Scott Gerson MD has been involved in Ayurvedic research for many years. As a qualified medical practitioner, he combines Ayurveda with conventional medicine in his New York practice.

The Health Essentials Series

There is a growing number of people who find themselves attracted to holistic or alternative therapies and natural approaches to maintaining optimum health and vitality. The *Health Essentials* series is designed to help the newcomer by presenting high quality introductions to all the main complementary health subjects. Each book presents all the essential information on each therapy, explaining what it is, how it works and what it can do for the reader. Advice is also given, where possible, on how to begin using the therapy at home, together with comprehensive lists of courses and classes available worldwide.

The *Health Essentials* titles are all written by practising experts in their fields. Exceptionally clear and concise, each text is supported by attractive illustrations.

Series Medical Consultant
Dr John Cosh MD, FRCP

In the same series

Acupressure by Richard Brennan
Acupuncture by Peter Mole
Alexander Technique by Richard Brennan
Aromatherapy by Christine Wildwood
Chi Kung by James MacRitchie
Chinese Medicine by Tom Williams
Colour Therapy by Pauline Wills
Flower Remedies by Christine Wildwood
Herbal Medicine by Vicki Pitman
Homeopathy by Peter Adams
Iridology by James and Sheelagh Colton
Kinesiology by Ann Holdway
Massage by Stewart Mitchell
Natural Beauty by Sidra Shaukat
Reflexology by Inge Dougans with Suzanne Ellis
Self-Hypnosis by Elaine Sheehan
Shiatsu by Elaine Liechti
Spiritual Healing by Jack Angelo
Vitamin Guide by Hasnain Walji

Health Essentials

AYURVEDA

The Ancient Indian
Healing Art

SCOTT GERSON MD

ELEMENT
Shaftesbury, Dorset • Boston, Massachusetts
Melbourne, Victoria

© Element Books Limited 1993
Text © Scott Gerson 1993

First published in Great Britain in 1993 by
Element Books Limited
Shaftesbury, Dorset SP7 8RF

Published in the USA in 1993 by
Element Books, Inc.
160 North Washington Street, Boston, MA 02114

Published in Australia in 1992 by
Element Books and distributed
by Penguin Australia Ltd
487 Maroondah Highway, Ringwood,
Victoria 3134

Reprinted March 1992
Reprinted January and August 1993
Reprinted 1994
Reprinted 1995
Reprinted January and May 1996

Reissued 1997
Reprinted 1998

Designed by Nancy Lawrence
Illustrations by David Gifford
Typeset in Goudy by Selectmove London
Printed and bound in Great Britain by
Biddles Ltd, Guildford and King's Lynn

British Library Cataloguing in Publication
data available

Library of Congress Cataloging in Publication Data
Gerson, Scott. Health Essentials
Ayurveda; the ancient Indian healing art / Scott Gerson Includes index
1. Medicine, Ayurvedic
I. Title II. Series
R606.G47 1993
615.5'3 dc20 93–36022

ISBN 1–86204–096–6

Note from the Publisher

Any information given in any book in the *Health Essentials* series is not intended to be taken as a replacement for medical advice. Any person with a condition requiring medical attention should consult a qualified medical practitioner or suitable therapist.

Contents

Acknowledgements   vii
Preface   1
1. What is Ayurveda?   3
2. History of Ayurveda   7
3. The Five Elements and the Tridosha Theory   13
4. Fundamental Concepts   33
5. The Disease Process   62
6. Treatment of Disease   77

Glossary   107
Useful Addresses   110
Further Reading   112
Index   113

Acknowledgements

Om Paramatmane Namah
A bow to the Supreme Spirit

Sincere thanks to my parents, Jacob and Doreen, and to my sister Nancy, for their love. Thanks from my heart also to all my teachers, tutors, and fellow travellers on the Path. Special gratitude to Dr Ashwin Barot and Dr Nicholas Kostopoulos for their support.

This book is dedicated to the memory of Thomas H. Griffiths whose spirit lives on in me.

Preface

FROM THE BEGINNING of human history, man has been engaged in the search for peace and prosperity. Excluding the ascetic, who has renounced all pleasures and comforts to lead a conscious life of privation and pain, nothing is to be gained from suffering and disease. The average person suffers, but involuntarily. The object of Ayurveda is to alleviate suffering and to preserve the health of the healthy and heal the diseases of the diseased.

Many people in the world today do not understand the real purpose of their lives. They remain enchanted by the material creation and lack any memory of our true divine nature. They squander their time and energy in selfish and thoughtless pursuits borne of fear and ignorance. This may perhaps seem a harsh view of civilization. However, this loss of memory of our true nature is at the core of many of our individual and planetary maladies. In the human being, the mind-body is the aspect which is subject to decay and disease. The pain and anxiety of its fragmentation and disorder are countered with love and attention in the hope of restoring cohesion and wholeness.

This art of restoring and preserving wholeness is central to Ayurvedic medicine. The ancient *rishis* (seers) and *sadhus* (saints) understood that for healthy mind-bodies to manifest we must remember and nurture the subtler aspects of our nature. We must align our lives, our thoughts, our behaviours with the interior, ageless, omniscient Self and then by his grace physical and mental health may ensue. The idea that the well-being of the manifest perceivable body depends for its existence on the unmanifest, unperceivable Self is foreign to the average modern mind. But

1

this indeed is the reality of our situation. In the Brihadaranyaka Upanishad, an ancient scripture, a sage declares: 'When the sun has set and the moon has set, and the fire has gone out, and the sound is hushed, what then is the light of Man? The Self indeed is his light.'

This small book will introduce the reader to many practical means of attaining a life of health, peace and prosperity. Used with reason and patience all of these therapeutic measures will inevitably lead to greater well-being. However, lest this point be lost in all the details which follow, let the true message of this book be sounded now, at the start. It is up to you, the reader, to hear.

The ancient sages have defined one supreme way to attain the final goal of a prosperous and happy long life free of misery. This way is through meditation. This is very simple and can be done by anyone, yet the effects are profound and direct. It has been said that anyone who meditates properly will receive all the benefits of every extant health system and spiritual teaching. Meditation is the key to unlocking and freeing human potentials otherwise condemned to wither and die. It is provided to mankind for self-realization. Therefore, if this book inspires nothing else, perhaps it will provide an incentive to implement this simple yet all-encompassing practice.

Om . . . Peace . . . Peace . . . Peace

1

What is Ayurveda?

We meditate upon the glorious splendour of the Vivifier divine.
May He himself illumine our minds.
Om

Rig Veda I,62:10

A YURVEDA IS A system of healing which evolved on the Indian subcontinent some 3000–5000 years ago. It was established by the same great ancient sages who produced India's original systems of meditation, yoga and astrology. Ayurveda has both a spiritual and a practical basis, the spiritual perspective engendering the practical. According to Ayurveda, humans consist of three bodies or aspects: the physical, the subtle and the causal. In modern Western language these could be referred to as body, mind and spirit. The Ayurvedic system of health care emphasizes that health is a harmonious functioning of all three parts of this trinity.

THE FIVE ELEMENTS

According to Ayurveda, everything in the material creation is composed of combinations of the five elements: space, air, fire, water and earth. These five elements derive from, and are the manifestations of, an unmanifest and undifferentiated Creative Principle, which is One. The five elements are not understood in a purely literal fashion, as in the fire of a candle or water

3

in a glass, but are rather meant to communicate the essential universal principle inherent in a particular element. Thus, air is the transparent, rarefied, kinetic force which sets the creation in motion. By fire is meant that force in nature that produces heat and radiates light. By water we understand the cohesive aspects of reality which hold things together, perfectly and simply witnessed in the ubiquitous H_2O molecule. Both earth and space are understood in the same prototypical sense. These five elements form the basis for all things found in the material creation, from the petals of a flower to the individual physiology of every human being. Balancing the elements is the key to maintaining health and treating illness, whether it be physical, mental or spiritual.

'Ayurveda' is a Sanskrit word which derives from two roots: *vid* which means knowledge and *ayus* which means daily living or life cycle. So Ayurveda is the knowledge of daily living and the life cycle. It is a medical system which emphasizes that all beings come out of nature, that we are an integral part of a whole universe and therefore have a responsibility to our source. It is a system which recognizes that the five elements come together in each individual in different combinations and proportions, making each person unique in their composition of elements, with their own path to balance. These differences need to be recognized and honoured, for if we live in ways which harm our bodies we are likely to suffer the consequences. Similarly, by living in a way which supports our unique constitution and in harmony with the environment, we will maintain health and well-being.

AYURVEDIC PRACTICE

The practice of Ayurvedic medicine includes eight branches or sub-specialities:

- General internal medicine
- General surgery
- Plastic surgery
- Otolaryngology (ear, nose, and throat)
- Toxicology
- Obstetrics and gynaecology

- Pediatrics
- Ophthalmology

In addition, the *vaidyas* (Ayurvedic physicians) are also familiar with the principles of nutrition, psychology, astrology, gem and colour therapy, herbal preparations and climatology. When viewed as a whole, Ayurveda represents an indisputable and dynamic model for those of us in search of an integrated and practical system of health care.

Healing ensues by the grace of the Absolute acting through the laws of Nature. All we can do is assist Nature by living a life of balance in accordance with her laws. The message of Ayurveda is to bring about harmony between the individual and Nature from which he or she arises.

The basis of all treatments in the Ayurvedic system is the balancing of the life energies within us. To this end it provides us with individualized daily regimens which deal with body, mind, and spirit. It uses meditation as a primary and fundamental tool, and also includes diets, herbs, mineral substances and aromas. It is as concerned with society as it is with the individual and seeks to give us the opportunity to understand and realize our true nature.

Ayurveda is often referred to as the 'science of life', a system of achieving and maintaining health. Health, however, is not the ultimate goal but rather a necessary condition for spiritual growth. The goal of life is not merely to live, but to realize the true significance of life. Those of us who are fortunate enough to enjoy good health should devote our energies to developing the highest of human qualities. Thus, while the body is not the goal of a life devoted to Truth, it is the foundation. For if health is lacking and troublesome, we may become distracted and limited in our ability ultimately to become detached from the body.

Ayurveda is a simple and graceful system of medicine. It does not offer a series of theoretical explanations to describe the way our human organism functions and malfunctions. On the contrary, it simply unfolds to the mind the laws of Nature. It instructs us to employ Nature's powers in simple and practical ways. It shows us that ultimately all power and intelligence flows from the Absolute. For this reason Ayurvedic wisdom was originally recorded in the language of the Absolute: Sanskrit. Like the Creation itself, the sounds, characters, and grammar of

5

this language are beautiful and peaceful in themselves. Sanskrit creates stillness within the mind because it reflects the stillness of the Absolute. Ayurveda also employs energetic principles which are simple yet profound and all-inclusive.

Ayurveda acknowledges the forces of nature which operate both within us and outside of us, and seeks to determine which force may be predominant in our particular physiology. For example, it can determine simply if there is excess water in the system, due to an imbalance of energies in the kidneys, rather than invoke complicated theoretical explanations of what modern medicine would term 'nephrotic syndrome', an arbitrary and unnecessarily materialistic term which conveys no practical information.

The concepts which are used in Ayurveda, by contrast, do not originate from scientific concepts or experiments, but come from *direct observation* of Nature. The five elements of Ayurveda, as we shall see later, are the powers of Nature itself operating within us and we are taught to observe and live in harmony with these powers. It is just as easy to become aware of these very same forces working within us on a physiological level. And so, just as being in water or being exposed to fire for excessive periods can harm us externally (by causing hypothermia or third-degree burns of the skin), allowing our inner water or fire to rise too much can cause internal dysfunction.

According to the wisdom of Ayurveda, the mind-body has the intelligence to heal itself. The same Intelligence which operates in the macrocosm – which governs the yearly migrations of birds, the changing of the seasons, the flow of the tides, the orbits of the planets – also operates at the level of the microcosm, the human physiology. It is the sole function of Ayurveda to promote the flow of this great Intelligence through each and every human being.

2

History of Ayurveda

In the beginning of Creation there was God, the Desire-Incarnate, imbued with the desire to create the universe. This desire was the first creative power of the Omniscient. The Desire-Incarnate and His great desire for creation were centered at the same place – the whole expanse of space. O Kama, shower riches and prosperity on the sacrificer.

Artharvaveda 12:2

THE CITY-STATES OF THE INDUS VALLEY

THE INDIA FROM which Ayurveda originated is largely unknown to us. What we do know is that the fertile Indus River valley provided life and nourishment for many city-states which existed between 3500 and 1500 BC. This was one of what are now considered to have been the five cradles of civilization: China, Egypt, Sumer, Peru and the Indus Valley. It is known that the Indian city-states of 4000 years ago were sophisticated and stable, encompassing areas between 400 and 500,000 square miles.

The fertile soil of the great river systems in this north-western part of what is now India made possible the production of surplus food. This led to the development of trade and, with the formation of cities, the beginning of urbanization. These cities were well organized and shared an intricate system of pictographic writing, standard systems of weights and measures, and well-thought-out building patterns. Two great cities, Mohenjodaro and Harappa were the centres of this great civilization, and their careful planning reflected a well-defined and coherent political order. They were serviced by an advanced system of sewers and drainage, and in general had a remarkably high standard of sanitation, which is reflected in the strong emphasis on hygiene found in the Ayurvedic literature. Homes were built of stone and brick and were constructed in such a way as to unify the entire city as well as to promote the flow of vital energy through the community.

It was an affluent, nature-oriented culture which worshipped the Mother Goddess. Like other civilizations of its time, large areas of land were allotted for the cultivation of cotton, as well as wheat and other grains. There was an active trade with Sumer, via the Persian Gulf and the Arabian Sea. Evidence has even been found of intricate clay children's toys, which further attests to the prosperity and insight of this early culture.

However, there are signs that this civilization was beginning to falter by 1700 BC, possibly because of a combination of invasions, climatic changes and shifts in the course of the Indus River.

Out of this sophisticated and evolving culture arose the knowledge of Ayurveda. The traditional lore of Ayurveda describes how the rishis, the wise sages of India, realized the necessity of removing themselves from their own civilization in order to find the stillness and clarity needed to receive the knowledge which they earnestly sought. Emerging from this thriving culture in the unspecified distant past a large group of rishis gathered in the foothills of the Himalayas to address the problem of disease and its effect on human life. Their object was to eliminate disease, not only from the human race, but from all creatures, and upon this they meditated together. It was out of these meditations that the understanding and information which was Ayurveda arose.

THE VEDA

The source of the Vedic tradition, which eventually gave rise to Ayurveda, is obscure but is thought to be related to the migration into the Indian subcontinent from the north-west of a people who spoke an Indo-European language, and who settled in the Indus Valley around 2000 BC. They are referred to in the Indian writings as 'Aryans', a term variously translated as itinerants or wanderers.

The Vedic Aryans brought with them religious concepts,

rituals, a consciousness-expanding potion called *soma* and a procession of naturalistic gods and goddesses. Some of these gods seem to have had counterparts in the religious traditions of the ancient Greeks, Romans and Persians, indicating a possible common prehistoric origin. The religion which the Aryans developed between 2000 and 500 BC was expressed in a collection of hymns and songs called the Veda (literally 'knowledge').

Hindus have always regarded the Veda as being of divine source and to have existed from all eternity, the rishis to whom the hymns are ascribed being merely inspired seers who received them directly from the Supreme Self. There are four texts which compose the Veda: the Rig Veda, the Yajur Veda, the Sama Veda and the Atharva Veda. Let us look briefly at each.

Rig Veda

The oldest of the Vedas, the Rig Veda consists of over 1000 hymns. All the other Vedas are based on it. Most aspects of Vedic science, such as yoga, meditation, mantra, and Ayurveda, are contained in the Rig Veda. Most scholars date it to around 1500 BC, although some contend that a much earlier date is indicated by archaeological evidence and astronomical references.

Sama Veda

The Sama Veda consists of various Rig Veda hymns put to a more musical chant. It is said to represent the ecstasy and bliss of Self-realization. While the Rig Veda is the step, the Sama Veda is the dance; the Rig Veda is the word, the Sama Veda the understanding.

Yajur Veda

This deals with the many yogic rituals and sacrifices for purifying the mind and awakening consciousness. The aim of these rites is to simulate the universe within the individual, and thereby unite the two.

Atharva Veda

Considered to be the last and latest of the four Vedas, this text contains chants and incantations to appease the gods and mantras to ward off evil, misfortune, enemies, and disease. Unlike the other Vedas, it contains magical spells used by the Atharvan priests.

Each of the four Vedas is divided into two distinct parts – the *mantra* containing prayer and praise to various aspects of the Absolute and the *brahmana* containing detailed directions for the ceremonies at which the mantras were used.

Also included in what is termed 'Vedic literature' are the texts which give secret and mystical explanations of the rituals, called aranyakas, and the Upanishads, the pinnacle of Vedantic philosophy, which can only be touched upon briefly here. Taken together, these treatises are known as *shruti* or received knowledge, as opposed to *smirti* (such as the Bhagavad Gita) which is remembered knowledge.

THE UPANISHADS

Towards the end of the Vedic period, the Vedic ideas of ritual and sacrifice were reinterpreted as being symbolic of an inner teaching. Speculations of a cosmological nature arose in various philosophical schools of the time; these were recorded and the treatises were collectively called Upanishads. In the Upanishads the spiritual meaning of the Vedic ritual and its relation to mankind are emphasized.

The basic teaching contained in the Upanishads may be gleaned from an examination of six great sayings (*mahavakyas*):

1. *Aham Brahmasmi*. I am Brahman.
   This establishes the identity of the individual with the Supreme Self. The Upanishads teach that our own Self is the presence of the Supreme Self within the heart.
2. *Ayam Atma Brahma*. The Self is Brahman.
   This states the unity of the individual Self with the Absolute; it also implies that it is the Self in all beings that is Absolute.
3. *Tat tvam asi*. Thou art that.
   Consciousness is everywhere and in everything and it is only the mind that throws up the illusion of 'other'.
4. *Prajnanam Brahma*. Intelligence is Brahman.
   This states that our individual intelligence is the presence of

10

Divine Intelligence within us, and through it we can realize the Absolute.

5. *Sarvam khalvidam Brahma*. All the universe is Brahman.
   That which is and that which is not is the One Supreme Self.
   Nothing else is, was, or ever will be except for Brahman.

6. *So'ham*. He am I.
   This reveals the Absolute in the natural cycle of our breath.
   So is the natural sound of inhalation, *ham* of exhalation.

In addition to the Vedic literature, there are many other secondary texts which are worthy of study and reverence, but which fall outside the aim of this present work to describe. Examples of these are the Puranas, the Ithihasas, and the Agamas.

THE ORIGINS OF AYURVEDIC MEDICINE

The body of Hindu literature pertaining to medicine and health is called 'Ayurveda': the science of long life. It has been suggested that Ayurveda is actually a minor Veda, a supporting or supplementary limb, especially of the Atharva Veda; other scholars dispute this view. But whatever their literary niche, these writings are counted as sacred. The earlier Vedic texts of about 1500–1200 BC were especially concerned with old age and various afflications, and prescribed cures involving prayer and herbal medicines. More importantly, the earlier Vedic view of the make-up of the human being is in agreement with later Ayurvedic descriptions.

The origin of Ayurvedic medical knowledge appears to be a combination of what has been directly received from a divine source and what has been remembered from the teachings of the ancient wise men. The Caraka Samhita, the primary and oldest known Ayurvedic text, begins with a gathering of great sages. The wisest and holiest men of the Indus Valley city-states, they had come together somewhere in the foothills of the Himalayas to address the problem of disease. They desired a disease-free society, not only for human beings but for all beings, so that the populace could observe their religious obligations and proceed toward Self-realization. So, as the story goes in the Caraka Samhita, the sages delegated Bhardwaja to go to Indra – a god who was knowledgeable about cures and remedies. Indra had received knowledge from the *ashwins* (heavenly physicians), who in turn had received it from Brahma himself. In the Sushruta Samhita, another important Ayurvedic text with a special emphasis on surgery, the source of knowledge is equally divine, although different from that indicated by Caraka. Here, Dhanvantari brings the knowledge back from the gods.

It can be seen that the Ayurvedic texts imply a connection between medical knowledge and philosophic thought and religious traditions – perhaps even an evolution from them.

CHRONOLOGY

BC	3000–1500	The Indus Valley civilization
	2500–1500	The migration of the Aryan people into India; composition of the earliest hymns of the Rig Veda
	1500–1200	Composition of the Rig Veda
	900	The Great War described in the Mahabharata
	900–800	Life of Patanjali, author of the Yoga Sutras
	850–500	Composition of the later Vedas
	850–750	Probable lifetime of Caraka
	600–500	Composition of the early Upanishads
	563–483	Life of the Buddha
	327–325	Invasion of India by Alexander of Macedon
AD	100–200	Rise of Buddhism; considered by some scholars to be the lifetime of Caraka
	400–500	Vatsayayana writes the Kama Sutra
	570–632	Life of the Prophet Muhammad
	600–700	Development of Tantricism
	788–820	Lifetime of Shankara
	800–1400	Procession of Islamic invasions
	1500–1600	Todarmalla composes the Ayurveda Saukhyam, a compilation of material from various authentic sources

3

The Five Elements and
the Tridosha Theory

From this Self, verily, space arose; from space, air; from air, fire; from fire, water; from water, earth; from earth, herbs; from herbs, food; from food, Man.

Taittiriya Upanishad 2:1

THE FIVE ELEMENTS

HUMANS HAVE FIVE sense organs and can therefore perceive the world in five distinct ways. The sense organs are the ears, the skin, the eyes, the tongue and the nose. Each of these sense organs is uniquely designed to perceive a particular form of external energy and to absorb it into the human body. The five energies or elements which are perceived by the five senses are known as the *pancha mahabhutas* or five elements. They are known by the following names:

- *Akasha* (ether)
- *Vayu* (air)
- *Tejas* (fire)
- *Jala* (water)
- *Prthivi* (earth)

It is important to recognize that the English translations do not and cannot express the true meaning of the original Sanskrit words. For example, by translating jala mahabhuta as 'water'

13

we do not mean to imply a mental image of ordinary drinking water in a glass. Rather it is the cohesive forces between the molecules and the inherent power of attraction in water which is the characteristic feature of jala mahabhuta.

The modern disciplines of physics and chemistry have organized the matter of the universe into many distinct elements. This has come to us in the form of the Periodic Table, taught in secondary schools around the world. In this table the elements are grouped according to their atomic weights, the number of electrons in their outer shells, and other objective criteria. All of these modern elements can be classified into the more practical categories of the five mahabhutas.

It is important to understand that although the mahabhutas are all uniquely distinct from one another, from another point of view they share many common attributes. For instance, the protons, neutrons, electrons, and other subatomic particles inside the atom represent prthivi (earth) mahabhuta. The forces which operate inside the atom which attract and hold the electrons in proximity to the nucleus represent jala (water) mahabhuta. The great energy which is released when the atom is smashed, and the latent energy present in its intact form, reflect the attributes of tejas (fire) mahabhuta. The force which moves the electrons around the nucleus demonstrates the dominant features of vayu (air) mahabhuta, and the space in which they move represents akasha mahabhuta. Thus, all five of the great elements exist in all forms of matter.

According to Ayurveda, in the beginning the world existed in an unmanifested state of pure consciousness. From that state of absolute consciousness, the vibrations of the first sound, the soundless sound Aum, began to manifest. It was from this vibration that the element ether was first born. Then, after some time, ether began to move and these subtle movements created the element air. The movement of the ether element produced friction and from that friction heat was created. From particles of this primary heat, light was formed which then generated the fire element. By means of the heat of fire, some parts of the ether were dissolved and liquefied, giving rise to the water element. Water element then solidified to form the molecules of earth element. Thus from the divine sound Aum, the ether was manifested, which then gave rise to the other four elements.

14

From the earth all organic and inorganic substances are derived, including those living beings in the vegetable kingdom, such as herbs, grains and trees, and those in the animal kingdom, including man. The earth also includes the inorganic forms that make up the mineral kingdom. Thus all matter in all of its diversity springs from the five elements.

The Five Elements

Element	(Mahabhuta)	Sense Organ	Sense	Elemental Qualities
Space	(akasha)	Hearing	Ears	Subtle sound, non-resistance, boundless, light
Air	(vayu)	Touch	Skin	Pressure, cold, rough, dry
Fire	(tejas)	Sight	Eyes	Heat, light, active, clear, acidic
Water	(jala)	Taste	Tongue	Liquid, cold, viscous, soft
Earth	(prthivi)	Smell	Nose	Solid, heavy, stable, slow, immobile

THE TRIDOSHA

All matter is composed of the five elements which are the building blocks of existence, but only living matter has the three *doshas*, or *tridosha*, the three forces which govern all biological processes. The term 'dosha' means 'that which darkens or causes things to decay', reflecting the fact that when out of balance, the doshas are the causative forces in the disease process. The names of the three doshas are *vata, pitta, and kapha*.

The doshas arise out of the five mahabhutas and can be regarded as the three primary energetic principles which regulate every physiological and psychological process in the living organism. From the most basic cellular process to the most complex aspects of biological functioning, the doshas regulate everything that occurs. The interplay among them determines the objective condition of the living being. A harmonious state of the three doshas creates balance in the physiology – in modern

15

terms, homeostasis – and this is the foundation of good health. Any imbalance in the tridosha manifests in a wide variety of signs and symptoms.

Each dosha is composed of two mahabhutas (elements) and from these elements each receives its specific character. The elements ether and air combine to form vata. Fire and water rule the formation of pitta, and water and earth kapha. Thus vata has the mobility of air and ether, pitta the energy of fire, and kapha the stability and solidity of earth.

Mahabhutic (Elemental) Composition of the Three Doshas

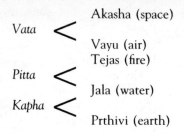

Vata stems from a Sanskrit word meaning 'that which moves things'; it is sometimes translated as 'wind'. It is the moving force behind the other two doshas, which are considered to be incapable of movement without it. It is responsible for all the body's activities and sensations. It is what channels perceptions through the appropriate sensory organs, converts them into psychological events and directs the appropriate response via the organs of action. It is responsible for the movement of air in and out of the lungs, blood through the circulatory system, and thoughts through the mind. It promotes mental balance and comprehension.

Pitta means 'that which digests things'. It is responsible for all chemical and metabolic transformations in the body, as well as for heat production. It also governs our ability to digest ideas and impressions and to perceive the true nature of reality. It stimulates the intellect and engenders the capacity for enthusiasm.

Kapha provides support and substance to the body. It comes from a word that means 'that which holds things together'. It structures everything from an individual cell to the musculo-skeletal frame. It gives strength and stability, both physical and psychological, and governs human emotions such as love, compassion, forgiveness, loyalty, and patience. Kapha can bestow resistance against disease and can support the healing process. Where vata and pitta effects are active in the body, kapha acts to restrict these two forces and prevent their excessive manifestation.

Qualities and Functions of the Three Doshas

Dosha	Qualities	Functions
Vata (space and air)	Moving Quick Light Dry Rough Clear Leads the other Doshas	Represents bodily functions concerned with movement. Controls the activities of the nervous system and the processes of elimination and respiration.
Pitta (fire and water)	Hot Sharp Light Penetrating Acidic Slightly oily	Represents bodily functions concerned with heat and metabolism. Governs digestion and perception.
Kapha (water and earth)	Solid Heavy Oily Cold Sweet Sticky Immobile Soft	Represents the structural aspects of the physiology and is responsible for biological strength, natural tissue resistance and proper body structure.

Together the three doshas govern all the activities of life: catabolism (vata), metabolism (pitta), and anabolism (kapha). When vata dosha is excessive there will therefore be excess catabolism, resulting in a breakdown or deterioration of the body's natural defences. Increases in kapha dosha result in increased rates of growth, weight gain, and a heightened ability of the body to repair tissues and organs. Excess pitta dosha results in disturbances of metabolism and heat production.

There have recently been some interesting attempts to find

modern allopathic correlations for the traditional Ayurvedic concept of the tridosha. It has been suggested, for example, that vata functions are all mediated through the release of neurotransmitters such as acetylcholine and serotonin, both in the central nervous system and at the muscarinic and nicotinic receptors of the parasympathetic nerves and the nerves supplying the striated muscle throughout the body. The actions of pitta have been compared with the actions of the sympathetic nervous system which primarily utilizes the catecholamines epinephrine and nor-epinephrine as well as dopamine to activate functions relating to energy release. Kapha action has been likened to that of histamine and the prostaglandins which regulate fluid balance in the tissues and control the permeability of capillaries throughout the body.

Although these analogies are intriguing they are, however, incomplete and not based on direct knowledge of the truth. They have been put forward by various scientists in India in an attempt to bring to Ayurveda the respect of the modern Western medical mind. Not only is such an attempt unnecessary, but the nature of Ayurvedic energetic concepts render it untranslatable into Western materialistic thinking.

The doshas pervade the entire body and mind and determine,

The Tridosha

Dosha	Quality		Physiological Action		Psychological Action
Vata	Subtle	Cold	Motor and sensory		Movement
	Moving	Rough	nerve functions		Creativity
	Dry	Quick	Respiration		Energy
	Light		Elimination		Activation
Pitta	Hot	Acidic	Digestion	Hunger	Desire
	Light	Clear	Thirst	Metabolism	Joy
	Penetrating		Vision		Memory
					Extroverted
Kapha	Solid	Immobile	Strength	Growth	Peace
	Heavy	Soft	Endurance	Regularity	Courage
	Oily		Lubrication		Friendship
					Generosity
					Tolerance
					Austerity

according to their relative proportions, the constitutional type of the individual. Individuals from each type differ from one another in their capacity for immunity from disease, their response to the environment, their emotional tendencies and their mental traits. We shall now examine each of the three doshas in greater detail.

Vata

Because it lends motion to the other two doshas, vata is considered to be the most influential. In the classical Ayurvedic texts, the functions related to vata all have something to do with movement, activity, vitality and breath. This follows logically from the fact that ether (akasha), which implies space and air (vayu) which is also understood as wind are the two elements which comprise vata. The tridosha determines the individual's constitutional type which reflects their predominant dosha; in turn, the predominant qualities of that dosha are most prominently expressed in that individual. However, to some extent everybody embodies all three doshas.

According to classical descriptions, vata people are either too tall or too short with thin, light physiques. The musculature is usually poorly developed, revealing prominent joints and bony contours. The hair is thin and often curly, the lashes are sparse and the eyes lack lustre. Their voices tire easily, sounding cracked and uncertain. They are hesitant and tend to procrastinate, lack confidence and are quite restless. They tend to loathe the cold, enjoy eating and prefer sweet, sour, and salty foods and hot drinks. Their urine production is not voluminous and the stools tend to be somewhat hard and dry. The skin too tends towards dryness. They tend to talk fast, interrupt often and walk noisily, and are said to have penetrating gazes. Sleep is often interrupted. Sexual needs are not strong.

Psychologically, these people are creative, alert and active. They learn quickly but have short memories. They have little willpower and tend to lack boldness and tolerance. Vata types are prone to anxiety, nervousness and fear.

We are not likely to encounter the sad prototypical individual described above, owing to the fact that, in reality, the pure vata type is modified by other doshas. In general the following qualities point towards a vata constitution:

- The body is thin.
- The skin is rough, dry, and cool.
- The teeth are large and crooked, and prone to decay.
- The eyes are small, dull, brown/black.
- Food is eaten quickly and is not thoroughly chewed; meal times and quantities of food are irregular.
- Memory is erratic; sleep is interrupted.
- Movements are restless and constant; they are unable to sit still; they bite their nails.
- There is a tendency towards hasty decisions.
- They are often dissatisfied with or unable to sustain friendships.
- Dreams contain images of flying, jumping, climbing, running and tall trees.

Ayurveda describes twenty basic qualities or attributes that characterize everything that exists in both the organic and the inorganic worlds. In Sanskrit, these qualities are called the twenty *gunas*. These will be discussed in greater detail in the next chapter. For now, let us note that vata has the following gunas, which it imparts to vata-type individuals:

- *Sita* – cooling, cold
- *Ruksha* – rough, dry
- *Laghu* – light
- *Sukshma* – fine, penetrating, subtle
- *Sara* – moveable, fluid
- *Khara* – raw, loose
- *Visada* – clear, transparent

Vata is described as both the driving force which initiates activity and keeps things flowing and as the main cause of most disruptions in the human physiology. Because it regulates the nervous processes involved in movement, emotions, thoughts, eating, drinking and our general functioning, its disturbances have very far-reaching consequences. It is easy to recognize an individual who has excess vata energy: the frame is emaciated, the skin dry and rough, and they may suffer from tremors, insomnia, weakness and headaches. They have irregular bowel movements or constipation, are unable to concentrate, have a decreased appetite, and feel insecure. The following table summarizes the characteristics of a balanced and unbalanced vata dosha:

Effect of Balanced Vata	Effect of Unbalanced Vata
Proper regulation of all bodily functions	Bodily functions impaired
Normal movements associated with eating, digestion and excretion	Movements for eating, digestion, and excretion inhibited
Mental activity controlled and precise	Mental inactivity and confusion; impaired memory
Control of the organs of perception and the organs of action	Perception and action are disturbed; senses are dulled, responses are slowed
Stimulation of digestive juices	Deficiency of digestive juices
Desire to lead an active life; vitality and natural interest	Loss of energy and joy for life
Normal drying of excessive discharges	Persistent bodily discharges
Normal respiratory function	Respiratory disorders
Normal sleep pattern	Insomnia, interrupted sleep
Excellent energy level	Non-specific fatigue, anxiety, worry, cold-intolerance, weakening of the Life Force

The classical seat of vata energy as a whole is in the colon. This is important when we attempt to treat vata-related conditions, most of which benefit from herbalized oil enema treatments in addition to other specific therapies. However, although the colon is the main seat of vata dosha it actually has five subdivisions, or sub-doshas, which are located in various centres of the body and which have specific functions. They are known as *prana* vata, *udana* vata, *samana* vata, *apana* vata and *vyana* vata.

Prana vata is the force for all the other vata sub-doshas. It is located chiefly in the head, brain and heart, with secondary sites in the chest, eyes, ears, nose and tongue. It is our individual parcel of Life Force given to us by the grace of the Atman. It determines our spirit and connects that spirit to the body and mind. It governs the mind and the senses. It regulates the functions of the heart and the lungs as well as the movements of swallowing, sneezing and expectoration. It is especially concerned with the ability of an individual to concentrate.

Udana vata means 'upward-moving air' and it is centred in the throat area; it regulates speech and exhalation, and creates vibrations of the vocal cords. It also functions to strengthen the memory and intellect and is said to determine our life's goals and aspirations. Stuttering and other speech defects are attributed to a vitiated udana vata.

Samana vata resides chiefly in the navel region as well as in the stomach and small intestines. It means 'equilibrating air' and is essential for normal digestion. The primary energies for digestion are actually the *agni* (digestive fire) and pachaka pitta (see p.25), but samana vata provides the air necessary for full combustion of the fire. It also assists in the assimilation of chyme and digested foods into the body.

Apana vata is focused in the colon but also resides in the bladder and genitalia. It means 'downward-moving air', and regulates urination, defaecation, menses, parturition and ejaculation. In addition, just as udana vata carries the life force upwards and supports the evolution of human consciousness, so apana vata carries it downwards and tends to limit consciousness. In practice, apana vata disturbances are very often at the root of vata disorders and need to be considered when initiating treatment.

Vyana vata means 'pervading air' and is centred in the heart, though it is distributed throughout the entire body. It governs the circulatory system and, importantly, is the aspect of vata which moves the pitta and kapha doshas in the human body.

Vata imbalances are by far the most common, and any number of factors can create them. Irregular eating habits, for example, can increase vata, as can foods with inappropriate tastes (*rasa*) as we will see in Chapter 5. In general, foods with bitter, pungent or astringent tastes will aggravate vata. Exposure to cold, wind, and dry climates will increase it, as will excessive physical exercise, frequent periods of hunger, violent behaviour, anxiety and prolonged periods of grief. The vata dosha is also known to govern the period of life from about sixty-four onwards.

Thus a vata-aggravated person can be recognized by a some-what anxious and unsteady demeanour, a tentative gait, a thin, somewhat dehydrated body, and a sullen, almost cyanotic skin colouration. In addition the voice may crack, and he or she may be unusually loquacious, interrupting often. As I have said, there may be an aversion to the cold and sudden decisions may be made without due consideration. If this picture is observed, a vata imbalance is certainly present. However, the picture is usually not so clear-cut because of the modifying influences of the other two doshas. Therefore the vaidya (Ayurvedic physician) normally begins with an eight-point examination. When vata is excessive the findings are generally as follows:

- The pulse (*nadi*) is thready, rapid and 'snake-like'.
- The face (*akriti*), namely the complexion, is darkened.
- The skin (*sparsa*) is cool, rough, dry and bluish in hue.
- The eyes (*drika*) lack lustre and moisture; the pupils are constricted.
- The tongue (*jihva*) is bluish with many furrows; the lips are dry.
- The voice (*shabda*) is cracked, rough and lacking force; there may be a dry cough.
- The urine (*mutra*) is dark yellow.
- The faeces (*malam*) are hard, dry and dark.

In contrast, reduced vata – a relatively uncommon condition – reveals itself in a decrease in the general activity of the body, increased lethargy, mild depression, and mental apathy. The specific types of diseases and treatment approaches to these conditions will be discussed in later chapters.

Pitta

Pitta dosha is frequently regarded as the fire within the body. However, this is not entirely accurate. It is more useful to identify it as the energy stored in the body as organic acids, hormones, enzymes and neurotransmitters. All of these substances cause the release of heat and energy as well as the breakdown of complex molecules.

The Charaka Samhita, a principal text of Ayurveda, identifies the main functions of pitta dosha as digestion, heat production, metabolism, providing colour to the blood, vision and skin lustre. In the realm of the mind, pitta produces brightness of the intellect, enthusiasm, contentment, courage and memory of the truth. In its purist manifestation a pitta-type individual would display the following characteristics:

- Medium frame and height, tending towards slender.
- Moderate muscular development; medium prominence of veins and tendons.
- Reddish or yellowish complexion; possibly moles, birthmarks and freckles.
- Smallish, sharp and often grey, brown, or green eyes.
- Hair tending to be scanty, greying early, and falling out easily, sometimes prematurely.
- A tendency to perspire freely.
- Moderate sexual desires.
- Sharp appetite; can consume large quantities of food.
- High intelligence; leaders, good speakers; tendency to be jealous, angry and judgemental.
- Openness to new ideas; heightened sense of responsibility; can make decisions and organize affairs.

Pitta has the following attributes which it derives from the mahabhutas tejas (fire) and jala (water):

- *Usna* (hot)
- *Sara* (mobile)
- *Tiksna* (sharp)
- *Drava* (fluid)
- *Snigdha* (viscous)

A person with excessive pitta may have a higher than normal body temperature caused by infection or inflammation, will be

24

thirsty, sweaty and fatigued, and will have a burning sensation throughout the body. The skin as well as the sclerae of the eyes may appear yellowish. There is a tendency towards anger, improper speech and foolishness. The following table lists the manifestations of balanced and unbalanced pitta dosha:

Effect of Balanced Pitta	Effect of Unbalanced Pitta
Strong and complete digestion	Poor digestion. Inefficient discrimination between nutrients and wastes
Normal heat and thirst mechanism	Irregular body temperature
Excellent vision	Impaired vision
Good complexion, generally healthy impression	Skin colour variable, inflamed, unhealthy; premature greying
Courageous, cheerful	Anxious, irritable, driven
Stimulated intellect	Dullness of reasoning faculty
Steadfast concentration on the truth; disciplined	Spiritually impoverished
Efficient assimilation of foods	Heartburn, peptic ulcer, irritable bowels, diarrhoea

Pitta's main site is the small intestines, and it also has five sub-doshas: *pachaka* pitta, *ranjaka* pitta, *sadhaka* pitta, *alochaka* pitta and *bhrajaka* pitta.

Pachaka pitta is the main energy source for digestion and manifests in the body as digestive enzymes (such as proteases, lipases, peptidases and hydrochloric acid. It separates nutritionally useful foods from those that are unuseable. It creates hunger and gives an individual a natural desire for foods which are needed.

Ranjaka pitta resides in the liver and its actions are in the liver, stomach and spleen. It gives colour to the blood, and is therefore the oxidative energy within the haemoglobin molecule. When an individual is physically or emotionally challenged ranjaka pitta rises and makes itself known in the stomach region. It can produce a fiery personality, give one the appearance of being red with rage, and cause gastritis and peptic ulcers.

Sadhaka pitta is the fire that is concerned with the intelligence, discrimination and clarity of thought. It is located in the heart. It is said to be the fire that forges the mind-body connection, allowing consciousness to permeate the physiology. It is also the energy that 'digests' concepts and ideas.

Alochaka pitta is located in the eyes and governs the sense of vision. If disturbed it can sometimes result in headaches.

Bhrajaka pitta gives a person a radiant complexion and its seat is the entire surface of the skin. When it is disturbed, individuals are prone to rashes and other non-specific discolourations of the skin. It is interesting that this sub-dosha is also said to govern our capacity for compassion.

Foods which are sour, salty and pungent will increase pitta; these include spicy foods, pepper, ginger, chili, cumin, yoghurt, lemon, vinegar and some cheeses and fruits. All these foods are heat-producing and mobile, and will serve to increase the rate of metabolic processes, stimulate endocrine secretions and create increased blood flow to particular regions of the body, including the small intestines and the kidneys. Overheating of the body and fiery emotions such as anger, aggravation and grief tend to augment pitta. Pitta is normally high between 10 am and 2 pm and again between 10 pm and 2 am. Its season of predominance is the summer and it is the dominating energy of life between the ages of approximately twenty-eight and sixty-three.

An aggravated pitta reveals itself easily by often causing fever and creating a yellowing of the skin, sclerae and urine. The faeces also tend to be light in colour and somewhat loose. Cold foods and liquids are favoured, and there is intense thirst and a burning sensation throughout the body. There is often generalized weakness, insomnia and skin rashes, and not infrequently there is an infectious or inflammatory process unfolding somewhere in the body. The eight-point diagnosis gives the following results when pitta is aggravated:

- The pulse (*nadi*) is of greater amplitude and fullness – 'like a frog jumping'.
- The face (*akriti*) shows struggle, discontent and anxiety.

26

- The skin (*sparsa*) is reddened, smooth, and warm; there is increased perspiration.
- The eyes (*drika*) are inflamed and icteric, with corkscrewing venules throughout the sclerae.
- The tongue (*jihva*) is beefy, red and moist.
- The voice (*shabda*) is forceful and heated; the volume is loud and the speech direct and rapid.
- The urine (*mutra*) is yellowish or reddish and hot and clear; there may be burning with urination.
- The faeces (*malam*) are loose and sometimes watery.

Reduced pitta, on the other hand, is manifested in a loss of the normal healthy lustre of the skin, a poor appetite, slow digestion and a loss of body heat. The specific diseases caused by a disturbed pitta dosha are fewer in number than those caused by vata. They will be described in a later chapter.

Kapha

Kapha dosha cements and gives structure to the body. The two basic elements of which it is composed are earth and water, and together these form a prototypical protoplasm – the fundamental stuff of life. Kapha means 'to keep together, to embrace; cohering'. It imparts to the mind-body stability, heaviness, firmness, strength, resilience and coolness. It provides the body with its resistance to disease and also gives great support to the healing process. Kapha is the anabolic force in the body and as such governs the formation of the smallest organic molecule or cell as well as the largest bones and muscles. It is supportive of those mental processes which are stabilizing and strengthening in nature: courage, vitality, loyalty, understanding, forgiveness, love and acceptance of situations as they are. Kapha's primary sites are the stomach and the chest. People who are predominantly kapha have strong, well-developed bodies with broad chests, supple musculature and healthy appearances. They do however have a tendency to carry excess weight. They are generally good-looking, with large charming eyes and abundant vital energy. The skin is soft and lustrous; the hair is thick, soft, dark, and often wavy. They tend to move slowly and deliberately. I can often identify a new patient as a kapha type by listening to his or her approach to my office door, which can sound like a running elephant! Physiologically, their appetites are regular and the digestion slow but steady. Stools tend to be regular or soft. They favour pungent, bitter and astringent foods. Sleep is *very* sound and long. They learn new things relatively slowly but, once acquired, knowledge is retained. Kapha characteristics can be summarized as follows:

- Strong, well-proportioned bodies with great endurance and integrity of the bones and muscles; a tendency towards being overweight.
- Large, calm attractive eyes.
- Thick, dark, wavy hair.
- Strong sexual desire and a capacity for sensual enjoyment in all forms.
- Regular and steady appetite and digestion; relatively small intake of food owing to efficient digestion.
- Intelligent thought, well-considered conclusions, clear speech; precise pronounciation; sweet, clear voice.
- Strong immune system; long life; not easily aggravated.

One of the functions of kapha is to restrict the excessive manifestations of the other two doshas. It owes its properties to the mahabhutas earth and water. The qualities associated with kapha are thus:

- *Guru* (heavy)
- *Snigdha* (viscous)
- *Picchila* (gelatinous)
- *Sita* (cold)
- *Sthula* (coarse)
- *Sthira* (stable)
- *Slaksma* (slimy)

In general, a kapha excess results in decreased body temperature, dullness, constipation, excessive sleep, obesity, weakness, goitre and a sweet taste in the mouth. There can also be decreased thirst, a white coating over the entire tongue, burning sensations and generalized urticaria with itching. The following table gives a description of findings when kapha is balanced or unbalanced:

Effect of *Balanced Kapha*	*Effect of* *Unbalanced Kapha*
Excellent nutritional status, firm musculature, strong bones	Poor nutritional status, thin, flabby
Adequate moisture and lubrication in the body	Dry; decreased mucus and saliva
Well-knit joints	Loose joints
Stable, compact and strong physique	Soft and weakened physique
Sexual potency	Sexual impotency
Calm, forgiving, understanding	Intolerant, insecure, jealous
Strong digestion	Slow digestion
Physiological moisture to the respiratory tissues	Excess production of mucus

The 'root' of kapha is the stomach and its main secondary sites are the upper chest region, the kidneys, the head and the joints. Like the other doshas, there are five kapha sub-doshas: *kledaka* kapha, *avalambaka* kapha, *bodhaka* kapha, *tarpaka* kapha and *slesaka* kapha.

Kledaka kapha provides internal lubrication for the proper digestion and absorption of food by governing the digestive enzymes and juices of the stomach, duodenum and remainder of the digestive tract. When it is deficient there is an 'empty' feeling in the abdomen; when functioning properly, a feeling of firmness and satisfaction.

Avalambaka kapha provides moisture for all the other bodily kaphas. It exists as the watery component of the plasma and is circulated throughout the body by the heart and lungs, which are its location.

Bodhaka kapha is located in the mouth and tongue and governs the sense of taste; it enables us to discriminate between the six basic tastes (sweet, sour, salty, pungent, bitter and astringent) and to recognize subtle flavours. The perception of taste is one of the initial stages of digestion, as it produces preparatory changes in the stomach and duodenum for proper transformation of particular types of food.

Tarpaka kapha, located in the head and cerebro-spinal fluid, lubricates and nourishes the brain and the sense organs. It also governs emotional equanimity, happiness and memory.

Slesaka kapha corresponds to the synovial fluids which lubricate and protect the joints, and it is also the principle which gives strength to the tendons and ligaments.

Excessive sleep, especially during the daytime, and overeating will cause kapha to become aggravated. Food taken before the previous meal is completely digested will have the same effect, as will insufficient physical exercise. Sweet, sour and salty foods also aggravate kapha, as well as cold and unctuous (oily) foods such as meat, fish, milk, yoghurt, cakes, and ice cream. Kapha is naturally high in the spring, during the first twenty-one years of life, between 6 am and 10 am and 6 pm and 10 pm, and one or two hours after a meal.

An increase in kapha dosha is indicated by sluggishness, exhaustion, chills, swelling, itching, stiffness and excessive exudation from the nose or ears. Other symptoms include a loss of gentleness and sweetness, whitening of the nails, pallor of the face, and a lightening of the urine and faeces. The eight-point examination will reveal the following when kapha dosha is exacerbated:

- The pulse (*nadi*) is regular, steady and slow like that of a swan on a lake.
- The face (*akriti*) shows calmness, even reaching detachment and apathy at times.
- The skin (*sparsa*) is pale, cold, soft and oily.
- The eyes (*drika*) have large brown irises with large white sclerae, and emanate charm.
- The tongue (*jihva*) is coated, whitish and thickened.
- The voice (*shabda*) is melodious, slow, soft and sweet.
- The urine (*mutra*) is cloudy and pale.
- The faeces (*malam*) are oily, thick, and light-coloured.

Decreased kapha can manifest as a slackness in the joints, increased thirst, insomnia, a rise in body temperature and mild constipation.

The diseases caused by kapha derangement and their respective treatments will be discussed in a later chapter.

It is difficult and at times almost impossible to translate the Ayurvedic philosophy, theory and methods into Western terms but in this Chapter I have made an effort to elucidate the concepts of the pancha mahabhutas and the tridosha. To the Ayurvedists, mere perception on the physical plane is insufficient for an understanding of the mysteries of life, and their system of medicine therefore embraces not only the physical aspect of life, but also the mental and spiritual. They recognize Man as a microcosm of the external macrocosm, with the processes of creation, maintenance and destruction identical at both scales. According to ancient Hindu lore, in the beginning heaven and earth were one; all was One. There was no space between heaven and earth for living beings to arise. Then by the power of the Divine Will, they were separated. In the space between the two firmaments manifested the Life Force which could support humans and all sentient beings. This Life Force became the five elements (pancha mahabhutas) and the three doshas which are at the heart of the Ayurvedic understanding of health.

The Three Doshas

Dosha	Effect of Balanced Dosha	Effect of Imbalanced Dosha
VATA	Mental alertness Proper formation of body tissues Normal elimination Sound sleep Sense of exhilaration	Restless mind Dry or rough skin Insomnia Constipation Common fatigue (non-specific cause) Tension headaches Cold intolerance Underweight Anxiety, worry Gastrointestinal gas
PITTA	Normal heat and thirst mechanisms Strong digestion Lustrous complexion Sharp intellect Discipline Courage Contentment	Rashes, inflammatory skin diseases Peptic ulcer, heartburn Irritable bowel syndrome Diarrhoea Visual difficulties Excessive body heat Premature greying or baldness Irritability Improper speech, foolishness
KAPHA	Muscular strength Vitality Stamina Strong immunity Stable joints Affection Courage Generosity Dignity Calm, mental tranquility	Obesity Slow digestion Sinus congestion Nasal allergies Asthma/bronchitis Oily skin Prolonged sleep Greed Attachment

4

Fundamental Concepts

I magnify God, as Agni, the divine Fire, the Priest, Minister of the sacrifice, Offerer of oblation, Supreme Giver of treasure.

Rig Veda I, 1:1

I N THE CHARAKA SAMHITA, one of the principal ancient treatises on Ayurveda, health is said to exist when all of the following conditions are present:

- When all three doshas (vata, pitta and kapha) are in perfect equilibrium.
- When all the *dhatus*, or tissues, of the body are functioning properly.
- When the three *malas*, or waste products, of the body (urine, faeces and perspiration) are produced and eliminated in normal quantity.
- When the *srotas*, or channels, of the body are unimpeded.
- When the *agni*, or digestive fire, is kindled and the appetite is good.
- When the five senses are functioning naturally.
- When the body, mind and consciousness are in harmony and the individual experiences bliss.

We have already seen how the tridosha theory, based on the five mahabhutas, is used to define balance for a given individual. In this chapter we will explore some of the other important Ayurvedic concepts which are essential to a full understanding of this healing system. We will start with the Sanskrit terms used in the above definition of health.

THE SAPTA DHATUS
(Seven Elemental Tissues)

The dhatus are the fundamental tissues which make up the body. Etymologically, the word 'dhatu' means 'that which enters into the formation of the body as a whole'. The dhatus are seven in number and each one is formed from the previous one, with the assistance of agni which provides the transformative energy required. The seven dhatus are:

- *Rasa* dhatu (plasma)
- *Rakta* dhatu (formed blood elements)
- *Mamsa* dhatu (muscle)
- *Meda* dhatu (fatty tissue)
- *Asthi* dhatu (bone and nervous tissues)
- *Majja* dhatu (bone marrow)
- *Sukra* dhatu (reproductive tissues)

Rasa Dhatu

When food is ingested it undergoes physical and biochemical catabolism until it becomes incorporated into the body as a tissue. The first stage of this process is the formation of a nutrient material called *ahara rasa*, which is neither food nor body tissue. We sometimes refer to this substance as chyme. With the help of agni, the digestive fire, ahara rasa is converted into rasa dhatu and the vata dosha circulates rasa dhatu throughout the entire body. Each of the seven dhatus is composed of all five of the mahabhutas (elements), with one mahabhuta predominating in each dhatu. In rasa dhatu, jala mahabhuta (water) is predominant. Rasa dhatu represents the plasma that contains nutrients from the digested foods and nourishes every cell in the body. Its condition is often reflected in a person's skin. If rasa is healthy, the skin has a glow, appears soft and smooth, and the body hairs are delicate but firmly rooted. The individual has an aura of vitality and a focused mind, and displays joy. Rasa dhatu can become unbalanced if the doshas become unbalanced. If it becomes excessive, there can be aching, nausea, heaviness, increased saliva with a bad taste in the mouth, and in general there are manifestations of increased kapha. A deficiency of rasa can result in cardiac arrhythmias, emaciation, hearing deficiency, thirst, weakness, impotence and depression.

Rakta Dhatu

Each dhatu has its own agni. Rasa agni helps transform rasa dhatu in to rakta dhatu, the second fundamental body tissue. Rakta dhatu corresponds to the formed elements of the blood: the white blood cells, the platelets, and especially the red blood cells. Some sources intimate that rakta dhatu has a particular connection with the haemoglobin within the red blood cells. The principal element in rakta dhatu is tejas (fire). Rakta functions to provide nourishment in the form of oxygen to the entire body. Healthy rakta dhatu can easily be recognized by evaluating the patient's lips, tongue, ears, hands, feet, nails and genitals, all of which should be reddish and plump to the touch. There is sensitivity towards the feelings of others, natural intelligence and a sense of enthusiasm. If rakta becomes excessive there may be redness of the eyes, skin or urine. The blood vessels typically become inflamed, giving rise to vasculitis, rashes and other skin conditions, abscesses, boils, jaundice, bleeding disorders, gout and irregular digestion. Deficient rakta leads to dry, rough skin, pallor and cold extremities.

Mamsa Dhatu

Mamsa dhatu has prthivi (earth) as its leading element; it corresponds to the muscular tissues of the body and it maintains the physical strength of the body and protects the internal organs. It is derived from rakta dhatu with the help of rakta agni.

It is the strength of this tissue and not its size that determines its quality. Muscles to be examined by the physician are those at the temples, around the eyes, down the neck, around the shoulders, the chest, the arms, the legs, and overlying the joints of the hands and feet. Healthy mamsa dhatu gives a sense of stability, steadfastness, community and strength to the individual. Excess mamsa dhatu gives rise to excess fatty tissue deposition and a sense of lethargy in the body; small fibrous tumours (generally benign in nature) are also common. Decreased mamsa dhatu leads to muscle wasting, weakness and an increased sense of fearfulness.

Meda Dhatu

Meda dhatu has jala (water) and prthivi (earth) as its main elements, and it corresponds to the fatty tissue. It is formed from mamsa dhatu. Meda dhatu provides lubrication for the body and gives the skin its slightly oily character. When balanced, it is responsible for the flexibility and suppleness of the body. The skin is soft, the voice sonorous and pleasing, the joints well lubricated. There is ample capacity for compassion, honesty and health. Increased meda is indicated by an increase in fatty tissue around the middle of the body and the breasts, as well as by decreased vitality and upper respiratory irritation. Reduced meda brings 'cracking' of the joints and atrophy of the abdomen, thighs and face; there can also be numbness and burning of the extremities.

Asthi Dhatu

Asthi dhatu is primarily composed of prthivi (earth) and vayu (air). This is reflected in the great strength of bone tissue despite its porous and light qualities. A healthy asthi dhatu manifests as strong bones, teeth, and nails; there are strong, well-developed joints and a strong skull. There is a natural enjoyment of life's activities, optimism and the ability to keep one's word. When excessive, asthi dhatu results in hypertrophied bony prominences of the skull and joints and prominent teeth. When deficient, the joints are often stiff and painful, the hair sparse and the teeth and nails brittle.

Majja Dhatu

Majja dhatu is nourished by asthi dhatu. Majja has jala (water) as its chief element and represents the bone marrow. Balanced

THE SAPTA DHATUS
(Seven Tissue Elements)

Dhatu	Mahabhuta	Healthy	Unhealthy
Rasa	Water	Lustrous skin Vitality Joy Focused mind	Heaviness Nausea Weakness Depression Bad taste in mouth
Rakta	Fire	Sensitivity Plump and reddish lips, genitals tongue, ears feet, nails	Inflamed vessels Abscesses Bleeding disorders Rashes Jaundice
Mamsa	Earth	Strength Stability Sense of community	Sarcomatous tumours Lethargy Fear
Meda	Water and earth	Lubrication Flexibility Sonorous voice Honesty	High fat Low vitality Numbness
Asthi	Earth and air	Strong bones, teeth, nails and joints Optimism Integrity	Joint stiffness Hair loss Tooth decay
Majja	Water	Resistance to infection Joy in movement Resonant voice	Bone pain Fatigue Joint pain Giddiness
Sukra	Water	Sexual desire Fertility Charisma Energy for spiritual pursuits	Obsessive sexual desire Dysmenorrhoea Low ejaculation Impotence Low vitality

majja dhatu gives resonance to the voice and suppleness to the body. There is also joy in movement and dance, and a strong immune response to infection. When aggravated, majja dhatu can result in chronic bone pain, bone infections (osteomyelitis) and chronic fatigue, while diminished majja leads to joint pains, fragile bones and excessive giddiness.

Sukra Dhatu

Majja, along with the dhatus which precede it in sequence, provides the nourishment for the seventh dhatu – sukra. This dhatu is the reproductive tissues of both sexes: the sperm in the male, the ovum in the female. Its basic element is jala (water). When healthy, it creates a strong sexual desire for the opposite sex, fertility and charisma. There is great happiness and energy available for physical and spiritual pursuits. When sukra is excessive, it increases the sexual desire to an unnatural, obsessive state, especially in males. Women may experience longer and heavier periods of menstruation, as well as spontaneous lactation in the absense of pregnancy and weight gain. Weak sukra dhatu leads to impotence, diminished ejaculation and testicular disorders in men. Women may suffer from metrorrhagia (irregular menses) and chronic fatigue. Both sexes may show symptoms of depression and decreased vitality, anaemia and a lack of interest in the opposite sex.

In the same way that one or two of the doshas may be predominant in a particular individual, the dhatus also express themselves in differing degrees. Knowledge of this fact can help an Ayurvedic physician in the treatment of specific patients. An often misunderstood point too is that the doshas, when in balance, are regarded as dhatus. It is only when they become disrupted that they become doshas (faults; that which darkens).

OJAS

Ayurveda understands the essence of the human being to be the One, the Creative Principle, the eternal, limitless Atman. Modern physicists might describe this indescribable force as the ultimate unified energy field which underlies all of creation. Ayurvedic physicians see humans simultaneously as energy and matter and view diseases in the same way. The seven dhatus therefore, while they are in one sense material manifestations, together form an energy within the body known as *ojas*. Ojas is the ultimate vital energy that is distilled from sukra dhatu and the other dhatus. It is the life energy that is located in the heart chakra and it pervades and enlivens the entire mind-body. It is said to be yellow in colour, transparent and liquid. When it is nourished, there is life; when it is destroyed, there is death. Where it is weakened in specific areas of the body, disease ensues; when it again becomes abundant, the mind-body heals. Ojas can be loosely compared to the fundamental energy of our immune systems, involving nervous, endocrine and psychological components. It is said to be similar in some respects to kapha dosha in that it supports and strengthens the physiology.

Ojas is produced through regular meditation, sexual moderation and avoidance of excessive stimulation of the senses. There are also certain herbs and foods which can help replenish it: milk, ghee (clarified butter), saffron, *ashwagandha* (*Withania somnifera*), *shatavari* (*Asparagus racemosus*) and many others. Factors which dissipate it include: anger, anxiety, excessive sorrow, worry, prolonged hunger, insufficient rest and excessive physical work. Additional factors which decrease ojas are excessive sexual activity, abuse of alcohol, stimulant medication, foods which are not fresh and an unsettled routine. It tends to decrease naturally with advancing age, and many geriatric diseases reflect low ojas, including senile dementia, osteoporosis and sensory deterioration. Deficient ojas can also result in premature aging. There are many modern diseases for which contemporary medical science can find no aetiology; these are often chronic, immune-related diseases such as sarcoidosis, Crohn's disease, ulcerative colitis, lupus erythematosus, cancer and acquired immunodeficiency syndrome (AIDS). It is very likely that these represent states of low ojas and may be approached therapeutically in entirely new ways.

MALAS

As a consequence of the foods which enter the body from the external world and the normal physiological processes which occur internally, we produce various kinds of waste materials, or malas. Faeces (*purisha*), urine (*mutra*), and perspiration (*sveda*) are the three primary malas and their proper formation and elimination is absolutely essential for optimal health.

Purisha

Each day approximately 8–9 litres of fluids enter the digestive tract. About 2 litres represent ingested fluids and the other 6–7 come from salivary, gastric, biliary, pancreatic and small intestinal secretions which are essential for proper digestion. Of this fluid, most is absorbed back into the body and only about 1 litre reaches the colon each day. The colon's principal function is to convert this liquid, which contains the nutrient-depleted dietary residue and cellular debris, into solid faeces for evacuation. Several important processes must occur in the colon and rectum for normal elimination of faeces to take place, including the reabsorption into the body of fluids and electrolytes, peristaltic movements which mix and help dry the faeces, and finally defaecation.

The most important element governing the elimination of faeces from the body is prthivi (earth). The most vital dosha is vata, which governs the various movements of the process, although all the doshas play a role. Any imbalance in the tridosha which manifests in an unhealthy condition of the faeces will be accompanied by predictable symptoms. Increased formation of faeces brings a feeling of heaviness and fullness, abdominal pain, flatulence, and borborygmi (gurgling sounds). Reduced faeces are associated with an upward movement of normally downward directed apana vata, with bloating, weakness and persistent dull upper abdominal pains. However, improper bowel function can not only create symptoms relating to the gastrointestinal tract, but also lead to disease in other areas of the body. Most notably, improper elimination can result in osteoarthritis, rheumatoid arthritis, bronchitis, asthma, sciatica, low back pain, dysmenorrhoea, headache and a variety of metabolic abnormalities such as hypokalemia (low potassium), hypercalcemia and hyperbilirubinemeia.

Mutra

Mutra (urine) is another mala whose elimination is vital for health. One of the functions of rasa dhatu and rakta dhatu, in coordination with vata dosha, is to carry wastes produced by the body's biological processes away from the tissues. The urinary system removes nitrogenous wastes, sodium, potassium, protein and bicarbonate from the body. This system also helps regulate fluid balance, affects the blood pressure and plays a role in the production of red blood cells. Urine formation begins in the colon where large amounts of fluids are resorbed. These fluids are transported to the kidneys (*vanksana*), where further alteration takes place before they are briefly stored in the urinary bladder and finally eliminated. The main elements of the urine are jala (water) and tejas (fire). Increased mutra results in polyuria (abnormally increased amounts of urine), urinary frequency, bladder disorders and infections, and kidney infections. Reduced mutra results in decreased production of urine, kidney stones, increased thirst, and abdominal pain.

Sveda

Sveda, or perspiration, has jala (water) as its primary element. It is a waste product which originates in the meda dhatu (fatty tissues). Perspiration helps regulate electrolyte balance in the body, has profound effects on the core body temperature, and sustains the normal bacterial flora of the skin in addition to removing watery wastes through the pores. Excessive sveda alters the bacterial flora of the skin and can lead to fungal infections such as tinea corporis (ringworm). There can also be an unpleasant body odour, itching, increased perspiration and decreased body temperature. Reduced sveda brings about dry skin, an inability to perspire, alopecia, a decreased sense of touch and burning sensations throughout the body.

The Three Malas

Mala	Increased	Decreased
Faeces (purisha) Mahabhuta: earth	Heaviness Abdominal pain Flatulence Borborygmi	Weakness Bloating Upper gastrointestinal pain Osteoarthritis Low back pain Asthma Potassium Calcium
Urine (mutra) Mahabhutas: water and fire	Polyuria Urinary frequency Bladder dysfunction and infections Renal infections	Reduced urine Kidney stones Increased thirst Abdominal pain
Perspiration (sveda) Mahabhuta: water	Fungal skin infections Body odour Itching High perspiration Low body temperature	Dry skin Low perspiration High body temperature Burning sensation

In addition to purisha, mutra and sveda there are other forms of bodily debris which are also considered as malas. These include exfoliated skin, hair, nails and ear cerumen. Since they do not produce disease, they are of less interest to our understanding of Ayurvedic principles.

SROTAS

Ayurveda describes various srotas or channels, which carry nutrients to the tissues and transport substances into and out of the body. When the flow of the proper substance through each channel is unimpeded, there is a state of health. When the flow through any of these channels is disturbed in some way (excessive, deficient or blocked), disease may result. The srotas share some of the characteristics of the tracts and systems acknowledged by conventional Western medicine, but they also conduct subtler energies which link mankind with the cosmos. Diseases in Ayurveda can be distinguished by knowing which srotas are affected, and by examining them through various diagnostic means the physician can come to know a great deal about the nature of the disease.

The Charaka Samhita describes thirteen srotas. The first three connect the human physiology with the external environment by bringing breath, food and water into the body. They are described below:

- Prana vaha srotas – channels bringing *prana*, the Life Force or vital air, into contact with the blood. This primarily represents the respiratory system and portions of the cardiac circulation.
  Site of origin: heart, thoracic cavity, abdominal cavity.
- Anna vaha srotas – channels transporting solid and liquid foods; the gastrointestinal tract.
  Site of origin: stomach, left side of the body.
- Udaka vaha srotas – channels transporting water. No Western equivalent.
  Site of origin: palate, pancreas.

Seven srotas supply nutrients to the tissues:

- Rasa vaha srotas – channels carrying plasma and lymph.
  Site of origin: heart, blood vessels.
- Rakta vaha srotas – channels carrying formed blood elements and haemoglobin in particular.
  Site of origin: liver and spleen.
- Mamsa vaha srotas – channels nourishing the muscle tissue.
  Site of origin: tendons, ligaments, skin.
- Meda vaha srotas – channels supplying nutrients for the formation of fatty tissues.
  Site of origin: kidneys, omentum.
- Asthi vaha srotas – channels which transport the nutrients for producing bone tissue.
  Site of origin: bone and adipose tissue.

- Majja vaha srotas – channels carrying materials for producing bone marrow.
  Site of origin: joints and bones.
- Sukra vaha srotas – channels carrying the sperm and ova and supplying nutrients for their formation.
  Site of origin: testicles and ovaries.

There are three channels which allow for the elimination of the malas (waste products) from the body:

- Purisha vaha srotas – channels that carry faeces out of the body.
  Site of origin: rectum and colon.
- Mutra vaha srotas – channels that carry urine out of the body.
  Site of origin: kidneys and bladder.
- Sveda vaha srotas – channels carrying perspiration out of the body.
  Site of origin: adipose tissue and hair follicles.

In addition to these, women require two additional conducting systems:

- Artava vaha srotas – channels which govern menstruation.
  Site of origin: uterus.
- Stanya vaha srotas – ducts carrying breast milk.
  Site of origin: breast and adipose tissues.

Some authorities consider the mind as an additional system, through which are carried thoughts, ideas, emotions and impressions. This system is termed mano vaha srotas, and it originates outside the body in the Universal Mind.

When there is free passage of the appropriate substance through each srotas, there is health. However sometimes one or more srotas can become impaired in some way and this can give rise to a diseased state. The Charaka Samhita describes specific factors which disturb or vitiate specific srotas.

- Prana vaha srotas (which carries Life Force) is vitiated by supression of natural urges, over-indulgence in dry foods, excessive fasting, doing strenuous exercise when hungry and performing *pranayama* (breath control exercises) without the guidance of a proper teacher.

- Udaka vaha srotas (which carries water) is vitiated by alcoholic beverages, prolonged thirst, excessive heat and astringent foods.
- Anna vaha srotas (which carries food) is vitiated by the intake of food before a previous meal has been digested, by consuming excessive quantities of food, and by improperly prepared foods.
- Rasa vaha srotas (which carries plasma) is vitiated by anxiety, worry and heavy, cold foods.
- Rakta vaha srotas (which carries haemoglobin) is vitiated by excessive heat, hot and irritant foods and excessive oils.
- Mamsa vaha srotas (which carries muscle tissue) is vitiated by sleep immediately following meals and an excess of the bitter taste.
- Meda vaha srotas (which carries adipose tissue) is vitiated by insufficient physical exercise, alcohol, excessive sleep and fatty foods.
- Asthi vaha srotas (which carries bone nutrients) is vitiated by dry, cold foods and sedentary habits.
- Majja vaha srotas (which carries bone marrow nutrients) is vitiated by traumatic injury, compression of the bone marrow and insufficient fat in the diet.
- Sukra vaha srotas (which carries sperm and ova) is vitiated by excessive or inappropriate sexual intercourse, suppression of sexual urges and selfish habits.
- Purisha vaha srotas (which carries faeces) is vitiated by suppression of the urge to defaecate and by excessive intake of food, especially when dry.
- Mutra vaha srotas (which carries urine) is vitiated by suppression of urination and by eating, drinking or having sexual intercourse while experiencing the urge to urinate.
- Sveda vaha srotas (which carries perspiration) is vitiated by excessive exercise, anger or heat.
- Artava vaha srotas (which carries menstrual flow) is vitiated by excessive aerobic exercise, irregular eating habits and mental stress.

- Stanya vaha srotas (which carries breast milk) is vitiated by fear, weight loss and emotional instability.

AGNI

Agni is the fire burning within us that kindles all the biological processes of life. Everything in us depends on it: our intelligence, understanding, awareness, health, energy, appearance, Life Force, core body temperature, auto-immune system, digestion – life itself.

One of the main functions of agni is to serve as the digestive fire and transform the foods we eat into assimilable forms. Many diseases arise from the improper functioning of our digestive systems, and this is often traceable to a disruption of agni. It is not only responsible for the breakdown of food substances, but also for destroying undesirable bacteria, viruses and toxins in the body which could impair our auto-immune systems. In the recognition, capture and eventual destruction of a foreign antigen by the body's own antibodies, it is agni that powers the cascade of steps to protect our lives.

In order to maintain and improve our health, it is essential that we nourish and care for agni so that it can properly transform our foods and provide nourishment for all the dhatus (tissues). When it is functioning well there is excellent digestion, normal elimination, good circulation, abundant energy, strong resistance to disease, a good complexion, a pleasant body odour and breath and an enthusiasm for life. When it is disturbed, however, digestion is incomplete, and the metabolism and physiology of the entire mind-body is impaired. Improperly digested foods form a toxin called *ama*, which then ferments and putrefies in the stomach and intestines. This gives rise to a poor complexion, offensive breath and body odour, constipation, intestinal gas, reduced vital energy, impaired circulation and a decreased ability to discriminate truth from untruth. Thus we see that, without exaggeration, the treatment of agni is a fundamental measure for most disease states.

There are thirteen forms of agni the most important of which is *jathara* agni, which presides over all the others. It rests in the region of the stomach and duodenum and catalyses the production of digestive enzymes and the initial stages of the digestion of all foods. It plays a major role in the transformation of foods into ahara rasa, from which all the dhatus arise and are sustained. Five additional agnis are called the *bhutagnis* and they are each responsible for the further digestion of one of the five basic elements (mahabhutas) contained in the ingested foods. They operate mainly in the liver. There are also seven *dhatu agnis* which are located in each of the seven dhatus of the body which regulate the physiological processes of each tissue.

The Ayurvedic scriptures mention specific factors which disrupt the functioning of agni. Among these are overeating, undereating, eating at inappropriate times, eating foods that lack nourishment and eating before the previous meal has been digested. Other factors are excessive sleep, excessive sexual activity, extremely hot or cold climates, anger, rage, prolonged bereavement, crowded or inhospitable living arrangements, acting contrary to accepted moral or social conduct and drastic changes in dietary habits.

Agnis are classified by Charaka into four categories, according to how they manifest in the human body: sharp, mild, regular and irregular. These four categories occur in the four primary types of individuals: vata (irregular), pitta (sharp), kapha (mild), and those with all three doshas in a balanced state (regular). Each type predisposes an individual towards certain characteristics:

- *Tiksnagni* (sharp) is usually seen in pitta individuals. Appetite is strong, as is the circulation and digestion, but impurities tend to accumulate in rasa and rakta dhatus. Diarrhoea is common. Immune status is good, but there is a tendency towards febrile and inflammatory disorders.
- *Mandagni* (mild) is usually seen in kapha types, who exhibit sluggish digestion, poor appetite, and yet a tendency towards excess body weight. Circulation may be slow, and although diseases are generally not severe, there is an increased incidence of congestion, bronchitis, influenza and common viral illnesses.
- *Visamagni* (irregular) predominates in vata individuals, who often display periods of intense hunger which then change to periods of almost complete loss of appetite. They often 'forget to eat' during their busy days. There can be intestinal

gas, distension, constipation or abdominal pains. Resistance to disease is irregular, and chronic and disabling diseases are more likely, especially those of the bones and nervous system.

- *Samagni* (regular) occurs not only in individuals of a tridoshic *prakriti* (their essential constitution), but also in individuals whose doshas are in a well-balanced state. There is a normal appetite, normal bowel movements, excellent energy and directness of speech.

Earlier we referred to the pitta dosha as the 'fire' in the body. The distinction between agni and pitta is an interesting one and is discussed at some length in the Charaka Samhita. The relationship between these two is analogous to that between a great general and his soldiers, or to that between the fire and the flame. The soldiers are the instrument by which the general acts; the flame is the instrument, the fire the underlying, all-powerful agent which holds the flame within itself. Thus pitta is the soldier and agni the general which gives fire, and thus life, to all metabolic processes throughout the body.

AMA

If agni becomes impaired as a result of one of the factors mentioned above or because of a vitiation of the tridosha, the first consequence is that the digestion will be significantly affected. Depending upon which bhutagni is most disturbed, certain food components will not be completely digested and will remain partially unassimilated. If jathara agni is affected none of the foods which are eaten will be completely digested. This mass of undigested food eventually accumulates in the colon, where it putrefies into a very sticky, white, foul-smelling substance. This substance is called *ama*. Ama initially forms and accumulates in the digestive tract but it can then enter other srotas (channels) such as the blood vessels, capillaries and lymphatics, where it can cause obstruction. In addition to grossly visible physical effects on the body, ama also has subtler consequences on the vital energies. If allowed to remain, it eventually undergoes further deterioration and produces toxic substances which circulate throughout the body via the srotas. These substances will accumulate in regions and tissues of the body in which the individual has a predilection for disease. There they reduce the body's natural mechanisms for maintaining the health of the tissues and create a blockage, contraction and loss of vital energy in that region. As a consequence a 'disease' condition becomes manifest after a time, and we then give it a name: gallstone, bronchitis, cancer, depression and so forth.

In Ayurveda two general forms of disease are recognized: *exogenous*, caused by factors originating outside the body, and *endogenous*, caused by factors inside the body. Ama is the root of all endogenous disease. When it accumulates in the digestive tract it can be diagnosed by examination of the tongue, which will exhibit a whitish coating. Depending upon the appearance of that coating and its location on the tongue, much can be learned about the degree of ama accumulation throughout the body. Ama is viewed, in Ayurveda, as the harbinger of misery, the cause of disease. The recommendation is to be relentless in our efforts to help the body rid itself of this venomous substance, and we shall hear about some practical measures for achieving this in Chapter 6.

PRAKRITI

As we have seen, the five gross elements of ether, air, fire, water and earth manifest in the human body as three fundamental irreducible principles known as the tridosha. From space and air comes vata, which governs our energies and movements. From fire and water comes pitta, which gives us warmth and the capacity to transform substances in our bodies, our bodily fire. From water and earth comes kapha, which makes up our structure, our flesh and secretions, the water in our bodies. Through the action of these three doshas, we replicate the great cosmic forces in our own bodies and participate in the eternal cosmic dance. Every individual has differing proportions of each dosha which accounts for differences in preferences, aversions, behavioural patterns and emotional predilections. The proportions of the three doshas present in any individual will determine his or her essential constitution, or *prakriti*. This essential constitution remains unchanged during the individual's lifetime and is genetically determined. It will manifest itself in us through our physical characteristics, natural urges, attractions and aversions, and psychological tendencies, as well as our development of the highest order of human qualities: love, compassion and evolution of consciousness. Thus the doshas are the very foundation of all aspects of man's existence.

From the Ayurvedic perspective, the first step in treatment is to determine the essential constitution of the individual. This depends on which dosha is predominant, and will reflect the energies and tendencies within.

The chart below is provided to help you determine your individual essential constitution. Individuals are combinations of all three doshas, with a predominance towards one or more. This chart is intended only to provide a starting point from which to determine you prakriti. As such, it should not be regarded as providing any definite conclusions. This should be done by consulting an Ayurvedic physician trained fully in Ayurvedic diagnosis and treatment.

DETERMINING YOUR PRAKRITI
Circle V for vata, P for pitta, and K for kapha.

Frame	V	Very tall, thin, very short, under-developed physique
	P	Medium, moderately developed physique
	K	Thick, large, broad, well-developed physique
Weight	V	Thin, prominent bones
	P	Moderate, good musculature
	K	Heavy, tends toward obesity
Complexion	V	Darkish, dull
	P	Red, ruddy
	K	Pale, whitish
Skin	V	Dry, rough, thin, cracked, flaky
	P	Warm, moist, oily, soft, moles, freckles, acne
	K	Thick, white, moist, cold, smooth
Hair	V	Dry, coarse, black, kinky, dark brown, curly
	P	Soft, fine, light brown, red, early grey or balding
	K	Abundant, thick, oily, wavy, medium to dark brown
Teeth	V	Crooked, large, protruding, receding gums
	P	Medium size, gums bleed easily, yellowish
	K	Large, white

Eyes	V	Small, dull, dry, brown, black, unsteady
	P	Sharp, penetrating, red sclerae, green, grey
	K	Big, attractive, charming, blue, white sclerae
Eyebrows	V	Thin, dry, firm
	P	Medium
	K	Thick, large, oily, firm, bushy
Nose	V	Thin, small, crooked
	P	Medium
	K	Thick, large, firm, oily
Lips	V	Thin, small, dry, unsteady, darkish
	P	Medium, soft, pink
	K	Thick, large, smooth, firm
Shoulders	V	Thin, small, down-sloping
	P	Medium
	K	Thick, broad, firm
Chest	V	Thin, narrow, under-developed
	P	Medium
	K	Thick, broad, over-developed
Arms	V	Thin, small, bony
	P	Medium
	K	Large, thick, long, well-developed
Hands	V	Small, dry, cool, well-lined, unsteady
	P	Medium, warm, pink, moist
	K	Large, thick, oily, cool, firm
Calves	V	Small, firm
	P	Loose, soft
	K	Firm, shapely, round
Feet	V	Small, dry, rough
	P	Medium, soft, pink
	K	Large, thick, solid
Joints	V	Thin, small, cracking
	P	Medium, soft, loose
	K	Large, thick, well-knit
Nails	V	Small, dry, rough, darkish
	P	Medium, pink, soft
	K	Large, thick, smooth, white, hard

Faeces	V	Tends constipation, gas, dry, hard
	P	Regular but tend towards diarrhoea, abundant, soft
	K	Regular, normal consistency, oily
Urine	V	Clear, scanty, frequent
	P	Abundant, yellow, red, burning
	K	Moderate, whitish, concentrated
Perspiration	V	Scanty, no odour
	P	Profuse, strong odour
	K	Moderate, cold, pleasant odour
Appetite	V	Irregular, erratic
	P	Strong, notices if a meal is missed
	K	Constant, can miss a meal comfortably
Voice	V	Weak, low, hoarse, vibrato, whinny
	P	Sharp, high-pitched
	K	Pleasant, deep, resonant
Speech	V	Talkative, fast, interrupts
	P	Precise, argumentative, convincing, sharp, laughing
	K	Slow, monotonous, low, harmonious, singing
Taste preference	V	Sweet, salty, heavy, oil
	P	Sweet, light, warm, bitter
	K	Dry, low-fat, sweet, spicy
Sleep	V	Interrupted, insomnia, 5–7 hours
	P	Sound, 6–8 hours
	K	Deep, difficulty waking
Memory	V	Short, forgets easily
	P	Average, clear
	K	Long
Emotional reaction to stress	V	Fear, worry, anxiety
	P	Anger, jealousy, irritable
	K	Complacent, steady, slow
Mental tendency	V	Questioning, theorizing
	P	Judging, discriminating
	K	Logical, stable
Dreams	V	Flying, running, fear, nightmares
	P	Anger, violence, sun, passionate
	K	Romantic, water, ocean, sentimental

Sex	V	Frequent desire, low energy
drive	P	Moderate, dominating, passionate
	K	Cyclical, infrequent, good energy, devoted

Financial	V	Spends quickly, poor, spends on trifles
behaviour	P	Spends moderately, spends on luxuries
	K	Saves, rich, spends on food

Gait	V	Quick, short steps, fast
	P	Stable, purposeful, medium
	K	Slow, stable, graceful

Weather	V	Cold, wind, dry
intolerance	P	Heat, sun
	K	Cold, damp

Disease	V	Nervous system diseases, pain, arthritis, mental
tendency		instability
	P	Febrile illness, infections, inflammations, skin
		disorders
	K	Respiratory diseases, asthma, oedema, obesity

Pulse	V	Rapid, thready, snake-like
	P	Bounding, strong, frog-like
	K	Slow, deep, swan-like

The letters(s) circled most frequently indicate which dosha or doshas are dominant in your prakriti.

GUNAS

Ayurveda recognizes that all organic and inorganic matter, as well as all thoughts, ideas, desires and actions have definite qualities or gunas. There are ten pairs of gunas, each consisting of a particular quality and its opposite – slow and fast, soft and hard, etc. The manifest universe can be seen as the play of two great antagonistic forces which continually create, sustain and destroy all that exists in the universe. These forces were called yin and yang by the ancient Chinese sages and *rajas* and *tamas* by the Hindu seers, who also describe a third balancing force, *sattwa*. Other traditions have other names. These two great complementary forces are indispensable to each other and cannot exist alone, like man and woman, day and night. Every substance on earth and in the universe is a manifestation of any number of the gunas which exist at the level of the unmanifest. The following chart lists these twenty gunas and briefly describes their actions with respect to the tridosha and the human physiology.

The Twenty Gunas and their Actions
(> = increases, < = decreases)

1. COLD (*shita*) > vata, kapha; < pitta. Creates contraction, numbness, decreased awareness, fear, dulled senses.

2. HOT (*ushna*) > pitta; < vata, kapha. Creates heat, anger, jealousy, expansion, promotes cleansing and digestion.

3. SOFT (*mrudu*) > pitta, kapha; < vata. Supports tranquillity, relaxation, love, freedom.

4. HARD (*kathina*) > vata, kapha; < pitta. Creates strength, support, discipline, contraction, duty.

5. OILY (*snigdha*) > pitta, kapha; < vata. Creates lubrication, wetness, strength, compassion, generosity.

6. DRY (*ruksha*) > vata; < pitta, kapha. Increases anxiety, constipation, contraction, slows tissue growth.

7. HEAVY (*guru*) > kapha; < vata, pitta. Promotes healing, body mass, increases lethargy, inertia.

8. LIGHT (*laghu*) > vata, pitta; < kapha. Creates awareness, movement, cleansing, happiness, digestion, lightness.

9. DULL (*manda*) > kapha; < vata, pitta. Creates relaxation, calmness, slow action.

10. SHARP (*tiksna*) > vata, pitta; < kapha. Promotes vision, comprehension, quickness, penetration.

11. SUBTLE (*sukshma*) > vata, pitta; < kapha. Creates lightness, penetration, motion, emotion.

12. GROSS (*sthula*) > kapha; < vata, pitta. Promotes heaviness, density, lack of understanding, ignorance.

13. SLIMY (*slaksma*) > pitta, kapha; < vata. Increases love, nourishment, absorption, smoothness.

14. ROUGH (*khara*) > vata; < pitta, kapha. Creates brittleness, indifference, dry skin, weakens digestion.

UNMOVING (*sthira*) > kapha; < vata, pitta. Promotes support, compactness, steadfastness, devotion, obstruction.

16. MOBILE (*chala*) > vata, pitta; < kapha. Creates motion, nervousness, instability, change.

17. TURBID (*picchila*) > kapha; < vata, pitta. Increases healing, stickiness, decreases clarity, perception.

18. TRANSPARENT (*visada*) > vata, pitta; < kapha. Promotes clarity, calmness, expansion.

19. SOLID (*sandra*) > kapha; < vata, pitta. Promotes density, compassion, resolution, loyalty, direct speech.

20. LIQUID (*drava*) > pitta, kapha; < vata. Promotes love, unity, compassion, digestion, absorption.

The doshas (vata, pitta and kapha) are each related to certain of these gunas as shown in the table on p.56. Foods, herbs or any substances with the same qualities will tend to increase that dosha and even aggravate it. For example, in summer the predominant qualities are hot, dry, penetrating and light – qualities which are similar to those of pitta. So by the law of like-increases-like, pitta will be aggravated in the summer. Likewise in autumn, the ruling qualities are windy (mobile), rough, dry, light and cold – qualities shared by vata, which tends to increase in the autumn season. In the same way kapha shares the qualities of cold, turbid, liquid, heavy and dull with the winter season and, as expected, kapha dosha in the human physiology tends to increase during this season. If one associates with substances which have qualities opposite to the ones which tend to become aggravated during a particular season, it is possible to prevent an excessive accumulation of the related dosha. This is one of the principles behind Ayurvedic preventive treatment programmes.

In order to comprehend the concept of the gunas fully, it is necessary to reflect deeply upon them. It is possible to understand them, however, if you observe the senses and the mind, for here much knowledge is available. Observe for instance what information the senses and the emotions give if one eats a generous portion of apple pie with vanilla ice cream. If the attention is on the body as a whole, one will immediately experience sensations of coolness, denseness, solidity and perhaps sleepiness, owing to the gunas shita, mrudu, guru, manda and sandra which are embodied in these particular food substances. Through an appreciation of these twenty gunas and their interactions, one can understand the basis of Ayurvedic diagnosis and treatment.

The Tridosha and their Gunas

Vata	Pitta	Kapha
Cold	Hot	Heavy
Dry	Soft	Cold
Light	Light	Dull
Subtle	Sharp	Oily
Rough	Liquid	Slimy
Mobile	Mobile	Unmoving
Hard	Subtle	Solid
Transparent		Turbid

RASA, VIRYA, VIPAKA AND PRABHAVA

The Ayurvedic understanding of herbs and food substances is based on a simple knowledge of energetics. Foods and herbs are organized according to their elemental composition, taste, heating or cooling effects, post-digestive effects and other unique qualities they may demonstrate. Using these criteria, the actions of many herbs and foods can easily be understood and therefore utilized in a precise manner according to the needs and constitution of the individual. A firm understanding of the energetics of foods and herbs is in fact essential for anyone wishing to engage in Ayurvedic healing.

Taste (Rasa)

The Sanskrit word for taste, *rasa*, is rich in meanings, all of which give an aspect of the importance of this concept in Ayurveda. Rasa means 'essential part, essence'. It also means 'sap', 'food juice', 'vital fluid' and 'elixir'. Thus rasa reflects the true qualities of a plant or food. It also means 'musical, artistic, lively', reflecting the enlivening effect of taste on the human physiology.

Taste, which is brought forth by the element water, stimulates our nervous system and affects all the systems of the body. Taste also enlivens prana and awakens the mind, and our vital energies are thus activated. Moreover, it is through the pleasing tastes of foods that agni is stimulated and proper digestion can take place. It is interesting to note that according to Ayurveda foods rich in nutrients may remain inert if they are poorly prepared and fail to stimulate agni. For without agni the power of digestion is lost.

Ayurveda describes six tastes in foods and herbal substances: sweet, sour, salty, pungent, bitter and astringent. Each is composed of two basic elements as shown below.

Rasa	*Mahabhutas (elements)*
Sweet	Earth and water
Salty	Fire and water
Sour	Earth and fire
Pungent	Fire and air
Bitter	Space and air
Astringent	Earth and air

The sweet taste is found in foods such as sugar, starches, cream, milk, ghee (clarified butter), butter, rice, wheat, grapes and some meats. This taste adds strength and also brings a mildly laxative and tonic effect. Salty refers to table or sea salt. It is stimulating, demulcent (soothing to the membranes) and laxative in effect. Sourness is represented by lemons, other citrus fruits, yoghurt, cheeses, vinegar and pickles. It is stimulating in effect. Spices such as black pepper, ginger, cumin, chili, mustard and cinnamon are pungent. This taste is diuretic, diaphoretic, stimulating and decongesting in effect. The bitter taste is found in foods like spinach and other leafy green vegetables, coffee, turmeric and herbs such as gentian, goldenseal, and neem. It is detoxifying, diuretic and alterative (restores normal function). Astringency is exemplified by most beans, persimmons, unripe bananas and herbs such as witch hazel, all of which have a contracting effect on the mind and bodily tissues. Thus astringent substances can stop bleeding and other excess secretions and discharges.

The Six Tastes and Some Common Examples

Sweet   Sugar, milk, butter, rice, breads, pasta
Sour   Yoghurt, lemon, cheese, vinegar
Salty   Sea salt
Pungent   Spicy foods, peppers, ginger, cumin
Bitter   Spinach, other green leafy vegetables, aubergines,
            turmeric
Astringent Beans, lentils, pomegranates, persimmons, honey

The doshas can be increased or decreased by various tastes. They are increased by tastes which have the same elemental composition as they do, and are decreased by tastes whose elements are opposite to their own. Thus vata (composed of space and air) is increased by pungent (fire and *air*), bitter (*space* and *air*), and astringent (earth and *air*), and is decreased by sweet (earth and water), sour (earth and fire), and salty (fire and water).

The following chart shows the effect on the doshas of *some* taste combinations, although many others exist in nature.

Taste	Doshic Effect
Sweet, sour, salty	> kapha, < vata
Pungent, bitter, astringent	> vata, < kapha
Sour, salty, pungent	> pitta
Sweet, bitter, astringent	< pitta

> = increases; < = decreases

When a disease state is present we often lose our sense of taste to some degree, and our appetite thus decreases and our agni is weakened. A weakened agni generally leads to an accumulation of ama and further advancement of the disease process. Therefore one way of improving agni and intercepting the disease process is by enlivening the sense of taste with appropriately chosen herbs and spices added to our foods. Food preparation plays a very important role in Ayurvedic treatments.

Potency (Virya)

Virya refers to the heating or cooling effect of a food or herb. Through this fundamental energetic quality, a substance will increase or decrease pitta dosha. There are three tastes which are heating and three which are cooling. These are listed in order of greatest to least potency in the following chart:

Virya

Heating	*Cooling*
Pungent	Sweet
Sour	Bitter
Salty	Astringent

Heating herbs have the ability to cause burning sensations, sweating, thirst, fatigue and digestive power. Cooling herbs are mentally refreshing, provide tone to the tissues and lubricate the srotas (channels).

Another factor to be considered in using foods and herbs is whether they are primarily drying or moistening. One of the chief qualities of vata is dryness, while kapha dosha is associated with moisture. Therefore tastes which are composed mainly of air (pungent, bitter and astringent) will be drying and will increase vata and decrease kapha. Those that are composed of water (sweet, sour and salty) will be moistening and will increase kapha and decrease vata. Pungent is the most drying of the six tastes, followed by bitter and then astringent. Sweet is the most moistening taste, followed by salty and then sour.

Yet another distinction is between the light and heavy qualities of a substance. Sweet is the heaviest taste followed by salty and then astringent; bitter is the lightest taste followed by pungent and then sour. Heavy tastes create substance and solidity in the body; light tastes promote weight loss and tend to stimulate the discriminatory function of the mind.

Post-Digestive Effect (Vipaka)

The six tastes of Ayurveda, after being digested and assimilated into the tissues, are reduced to three post-digestive final tastes, or *vipakas*. Sweet and salty substances have a sweet vipaka, sour substances have a sour vipaka, and pungent, bitter, and astringent substances have a pungent vipaka.

If substances are consumed over long periods of time, they tend to aggravate the dosha whose vipaka they possess. Thus pungent, bitter and astringent foods tend to increase dryness in the colon and vitiate vata. Sour foods will stimulate gastric acids, bile, trypsin and other digestive enzymes and thus aggravate pitta. Sweet and salty substances will create an increase in saliva and other kapha secretions. In general, pungent vipaka leads to intestinal gas and constipation. It also decreases production of semen and genital secretions. Sweet vipaka promotes the formation of all bodily secretions. The vipaka of a substance provides another useful context in which to understand the effects of foods and herbs on the human physiology.

Unique Energy (Prabhava)

Rasa, virya, and vipaka provide an excellent system to understand the properties of foods and herbs in most cases. However, some substances have effects on the human organism which are not predictable from a knowledge of energetics and fall outside the system. This too was recognized by the ancient Ayurvedic sages. The unique energies contained within a food or herb which defy logic and science are given the name *prabhava*.

It should be remembered that Ayurveda is not limited by any materialistic or dualistic paradigm of thought and that it fully embraces the mystical and spiritual aspects of all substances in creation. The systems which are elucidated in this book, including the mahabhutas, tridosha, rasa, prabhava and the rest, are meant to be guides for our understanding, not fixed laws. Therefore, one aspect of prabhava is the ability of certain plant products to affect the mind and powers of perception, sometimes giving rise to a more direct connection with reality.

One common example of prabhava is found in the mylobalan fruit known as *amla (Embelica officinalis)*. Amla means 'sour' and this fruit would certainly be expected to have a heating virya.

Yet not only is amla cooling, but it is also known to possess great rejuvenating and vitalizing properties. These properties are completely inconsistent with the energetic make-up of this fruit. This is prabhava. When using Ayurvedic principles to promote healing with substances provided by the earth, we must always keep our minds open to the subtle forces which may be operating beyond our comprehension.

5

The Disease Process

Untrammeled in the midst of men, the Earth, adorned with heights and gentle slopes and plains, bears plants and herbs of various healing powers. May she spread wide for us and afford us joy.

Artharvaveda 12:2

BOTH MODERN AND AYURVEDIC medicine seek to maintain the well-being of society and to prevent illness. However the current medical paradigm of health and illness suffers from a fundamental barrier to understanding the true nature of the healing process. Modern Western medicine proceeds from the notion that the mind and body are separate entities and that the body is the only appropriate arena for medical treatment, while the mind is the arena for psychological therapies. The entities are seen as separate and without a significant effect on each other.

There are two disturbing consequences of this attitude. The first is that there is no recognition of the spirit of the individual; the second is that it ignores the undeniable connection of each individual with other people and with the energies which surround us in the 'outside' environment. Ayurvedic medicine, on the other hand, views the individual as a complex whole consisting of body-mind-spirit, which is intimately connected to the environment.

These two radically different understandings of the human organism have caused the two systems to proceed in different directions. Modern medicine concerns itself with individual categories of disease which are distinct from each other and can be named. It focuses exclusively upon that disease and finds the agent or agents responsible for it, and then attempts to change or destroy that agent. A simple example might be someone who goes to an allopathic doctor with a persistent and painful cough accompanied by a high fever. The doctor would perform a sputum culture and a chest X-ray, and would perhaps conclude that the individual was suffering from a disease known as 'pneumonia' caused by a pathological agent called *Pseudomonas aeruginosa*. Allopathic practitioners start with several isolated symptoms, give them a label (the name of a specific disease), and then seek a specific *cause* for a specific *disease*. They then employ a specific form of treatment, usually a synthetic pharmaceutical product, to eradicate the aggravating agent from the body. The disease may actually affect various parts of the mind and body, but the modern physician is trained to view it as a localized, self-contained event. By naming the event with a diagnostic term ('pneumonia') the doctor narrows down the frame of reference from the whole person to an isolated part.

In contrast, the Ayurvedic physician looks at the complete individual, with a view of the entire body, the mind, the spirit and the environment. All information from these four realms is deemed relevant, along with the overt symptoms. This information is gathered and interwoven along with the person's other natural characteristics until it forms what is known in Ayurveda as prakriti, the individual's unique constitutional type. Overlying this constitutional type, the Ayurvedic physician can determine any patterns of imbalance which may be present. Thus Ayurvedic medicine does not identify a specific disease or a specific cause, but gives instead an integrated description of the whole individual. Ayurveda is primarily concerned with relationships between different processes occurring simultaneously. The issue of what specific cause is responsible for what specific effect is secondary to the general pattern of events. Ayurvedic medicine synthesizes and organizes signs and symptoms into understandable patterns which in the healthy state are in harmony. Any disharmony can be witnessed and the therapies seek to restore harmony to the entire pattern, which is the individual. A symptom is not traced back to a specific cause, but is instead viewed as part of a total pattern. Ayurvedic medicine, therefore, is holistic – embracing the truth that no individual part can be understood except in its relation to the whole.

Earlier we defined the state of health according to Ayurveda as the presence of all of the following conditions: the doshas are all in balance, agni is functioning normally, the malas are being produced and eliminated efficiently, the five senses are functioning normally and there is harmony among the body, mind and spirit. As we proceed with our discussion of disease it would be useful to keep this definition of health in mind.

All diseases which arise in the human physiology can be classified generally into three types: vata (space and air), pitta (fire and water) and kapha (water and earth), according to the predominant way in which the disease presents itself. For example, the presence of a severe sore throat, generalized erythematous rash, and a fever ('measles') would indicate a disease of a pitta nature. The presentation of a cough productive of copious amounts of whitish secretions, mildly swollen glands, with no fever ('bronchitis') would indicate a predominantly kapha condition. Thus all diseases manifest the dosha which produces them and we can understand the nature of any disease according to the kinds of qualities reflected in the mind and body. Although some diseases are produced by combined imbalances in two or more doshas, most have a predominant dosha associated with them. It is interesting to note that the majority of the diseases of mankind are vata in nature. Ayurvedic sources describe eighty vata, forty pitta, and twenty kapha diseases.

Vata diseases (space and air) include most disorders of the nervous system, headaches, insomnia, paralysis, epilepsy, constipation and arthritis. They display abnormal movements of the body's energies, pain, atrophy of the tissues, coldness and dryness.

Pitta diseases (fire and water) include most fever-producing states, blood dyscrasias, liver and gall-bladder diseases, ulcers, hyperacidity, skin disorders and inflammatory processes throughout the body. These conditions all display heat, rubor, moisture and movement.

Kapha diseases include most renal disorders as well as many respiratory diseases such as asthma, influenza, bronchitis, lymphadenitis, tumours, sinusitis and oedema. Kapha diseases display moisture, aberrant tissue growth, oiliness, and coldness.

General Disease Categories
of the Tridosha

Vata	Pitta	Kapha
Nervous tissue	Fevers	Respiratory
Tissue atrophy	Blood dyscrasias	(asthma,
Headaches	Liver/gall-bladder	bronchitis,
Insomnia	Ulcers	influenza)
Constipation	Hyperacidity	Renal
Paralysis	Skin	Sinusitis
Weakness	Inflammatory	Oedema
Arthritis	diseases	Tumours
Dryness		Lymphadenitis
Abnormal movements		Abnormal growth
		and secretion

The following lists give the diseases produced by aggravation of each of the three doshas. Diseases are produced primarily by *aggravated* doshas; depleted doshas are regarded as secondary reactions to other aggravated doshas and are incapable in themselves of giving rise to disease. The Ayurvedic diseases are accompanied by the corresponding allopathic name only so that the reader can to some degree understand the imbalance indicated. Sometimes the Sanskrit term has a remarkably current medical translation, while other terms can only be inadequately described in English. Remember that the Sanskrit terms are rich in meaning and indicate a set of unique imbalances in the body, mind and spirit; they are not merely names of diseases. Furthermore, this is the original list compiled in the Charaka Samhita. Many more diseases have now been described – in fact every disease state that could possibly arise in the human race can be understood in terms of the universal principles of Ayurveda.

DISEASES OF THE THREE DOSHAS

Vata Diseases

1. Nakhabheda (cracking of the nails)
2. Vipadika (cracking of the feet)
3. Padasula (pain in the feet)

4. Padabhramsa (foot drop)
5. Padasuptata (numbness of the feet)
6. Vatakhuddata (club foot)
7. Gulphagraha (stiff ankle)
8. Pindikodvestana (cramp in the calf)
9. Grdhrasi (sciatica)
10. Janubheda (genu verum)
11. Januvislesa (genu valgam)
12. Urustambha (stiffness of the thigh)
13. Urusada (thigh pain)
14. Pangulya (paraplegia)
15. Gudabhramsa (rectal prolapse)
16. Gudarti (tenesmus)
17. Vrsanaksepa (scrotal pain)
18. Sephastambha (priapism)
19. Vanksananaha (groin tension)
20. Sronibheda (pelvic girdle pain)
21. Vidbheda (diarrhoea)
22. Udavarta (increased peristalsis)
23. Khanjatva (lameness)
24. Kubjatva (kyphosis)
25. Vamanatva (dwarfism)
26. Trikagraha (sacroiliac arthritis)
27. Prsthagraha (back stiffness)
28. Parsvavamarda (chest pain)
29. Udaravesta (griping abdominal pain)
30. Hrnmoha (bradycardia)
31. Hrddrava (tachycardia)
32. Vaksa uddharsa (friction pain in the chest)
33. Vaksa uparodha (diminished thoracic excursions)
34. Vaksastoda (stabbing pain in the chest)
35. Bahusosa (arm atrophy)
36. Grivastambha (stiff neck)
37. Manyastambha (torticollis)
38. Kanthoddhvamsa (hoarseness)
39. Hanubheda (temporomandibular joint pain)
40. Osthabheda (lip pain)
41. Aksibheda (eye pain)
42. Dantabheda (toothache)
43. Dantasaithilya (loose teeth)
44. Mukatva (aphasia)

45. Vaksanga (slow speech)
46. Kasayasyata (astringent taste in the mouth)
47. Mukhasosa (dry mouth)
48. Arasajnata (ageusia)
49. Ghrananasa (anosmia)
50. Karnasula (earache)
51. Asabdasravana (tinnitus)
52. Uccaihsruti (deafness)
53. Badhirya (hearing loss)
54. Vartmastambha (ptosis)
55. Vartmasankoca (entropion)
56. Timira (cataract)
57. Aksisula (pinching pain in the eye)
58. Aksivyudasa (sunken eyeball)
59. Sankhabheda (temporal pain)
60. Lalatabheda (frontal pain)
61. Bhruvyudasa (drooping of the eyelid)
62. Siroruk (headache)
63. Kesabhumisphutana (dandruff)
64. Ardita (facial palsy)
65. Ekangaroga (monoplegia)
66. Sarvangaroga (polyplegia)
67. Paksavadha (hemiplegia)
68. Aksepaka (clonic convulsion)
69. Dandaka (tonic convulsion)
70. Tama (fainting)
71. Bhrama (giddiness)
72. Vepathu (tremor)
73. Jrmbha (yawning)
74. Hikka (hiccups)
75. Vissada (asthenia)
76. Atipralapa (delirium)
77. Rauksa parusya (dryness and hardness)
78. Asvapna (sleeplessness)
79. Syavarunavabhasta (red appearance)
80. Anavasthitacittatva (mental instability)

Pitta Diseases

1. Osa (heat)
2. Plosa (scorching)

3. Daha (burning)
4. Davathu (boiling)
5. Dhumaka (fuming)
6. Amlaka (acid eructation)
7. Vidaha (burning sensation of the chest)
8. Antardaha (burning sensation of the body)
9. Amsadaha (burning sensation of the shoulder)
10. Usmadhikya (high temperature)
11. Atisveda (excessive perspiring)
12. Angagandha (foul body odour)
13. Angavadarana (cracking pain of the body)
14. Sonitakleda (slowing of the blood flow)
15. Mamsakleda (muscle fatigue)
16. Tvagdaha (burning sensation of the skin)
17. Tvagavadarana (cracking of the skin)
18. Carmadalana (itching of the skin)
19. Raktakostha (urticaria)
20. Raktavisphota (red vesicle)
21. Rakta pitta (tendency to bleeding)
22. Raktamandala (red wheals)
23. Haritatva (greenishness)
24. Haridratva (icterus)
25. Nilika (blue nevi)
26. Kaksa (herpes genitalis)
27. Kamala (jaundice)
28. Tiktasyata (bitter taste)
29. Lohitagandhasyata (smell of blood from the mouth)
30. Putimukhata (foul odour of the mouth)
31. Trsnadhikya (excessive thirst)
32. Atrpti (non-satisfaction)
33. Asyavipaka (stomatitis)
34. Galapaka (pharyngitis)
35. Aksipaka (conjunctivitis)
36. Gudapaka (proctitis)
37. Medhrapaka (inflammation of the penis)
38. Jivadana (haemorrhage)
39. Tamahpravesa (fainting)
40. Haritaharidra netra, mutra, varcastva (greenish-yellow colouration of the eyes, urine, faeces)

Kapha Diseases

1. Trpti (anorexia nervosa)
2. Tandra (drowsiness)
3. Nidradhikya (excessive sleep)
4. Staimitya (timidity)
5. Gurugatrata (heaviness)
6. Alasya (laziness)
7. Mukhamadhurya (sweet taste)
8. Mukhasrava (salivation)
9. Slesmodgirana (excessive mucus production)
10. Maladhikya (excess bodily excretion)
11. Balasada (loss of strength)
12. Apakti (indigestion)
13. Hrdayopalepa (mucus around the heart)
14. Kanthopalepa (mucus in the throat)
15. Dhamanipraticaya (atherosclerosis)
16. Atisthaulya (obesity)
17. Galaganda (goitre)
18. Sitagnitva (diminished digestion)
19. Udarda (urticaria)
20. Svetarabhasata (pallor)

Although diseases are generally associated with one aggravated dosha, many may arise from an excess of *any* of the three doshas. For example, diarrhoea can occur as a result of high vata, high pitta or high kapha dosha. In order to understand this idea we must remember that the doshas, when aggravated, tend to disrupt each other. As the fundamental energies governing the functions of the mind and body, not only can they cause disease, but they are the location at which disease occurs. Because each dosha is associated with different organs and tissues, diseases of these organs and tissues will result in a vitiation (disruption) of that dosha. Hence, diseases of the respiratory system will reveal kapha as the location of the imbalance, and in general they will usually show a kapha imbalance. However, they may also have vata and pitta imbalances as their aetiology, because these doshas, when sufficiently vitiated, can disrupt kapha dosha. For example, high vata, having affected the vocal cords and caused hoarseness, may then create a disturbance of the mucus-secreting glands which line the bronchi, resulting in an exacerbation of bronchial asthma – which would reveal itself as a kapha excess. The doshas thus affect each other, and in very severe diseases, such as HIV-related conditions, all three may be vitiated, rendering treatment problematic.

THREE CAUSES OF DISEASE

When the tridosha (the three doshas as a single harmonious system) becomes unbalanced, disease in some form will manifest. What causes the doshas to become unbalanced is the cause of disease. There are said to be three factors which lead to imbalance of the doshas:

Misuse of the Mind and Body (Prajnaparadha)

This category includes all thoughts or actions which breach the natural order of human life and cause impairment of the intellect, emotions and memory. This includes, but is not limited to: the suppression of any natural urges such as coughing, sneezing, defaecation or urination; the excessive stimulation of natural urges; overindulgence in sexual activity; the incorrect use of therapies, starting therapies at improper times; non-use of therapies; poor conduct, immodest behaviour; lack of respect for teachers and elders; enjoyment of harmful objects; enjoyment of activities which cause madness; using inappropriate force; friendship with persons who commit evil actions; neglect of healthy activities; anger; fear; greed; vanity; hatred; intoxication; not speaking the truth; selfish acts; and disregard of local customs.

Unhealthy Association of the Sense Organs with Sense Objects (Asatmyendriyartha Samyoga)

This category includes over- under- and non-stimulation of the five sense organs. As far as the eyes are concerned, this includes gazing excessively at very bright objects, holding objects too far from or too close to the eyes, seeing things that are deformed, alarming, agitating, terrifying, shocking or contemptuous, and not using the eyes at all.

As regards hearing, it includes loud, thunderous noises, piercing cries, grieving cries, harsh language, news of the death of friends or family, and insulting, assaulting or untruthful sounds.

Excessive utilization of smell would include any intoxicating, strong, sharp odours; wrong use would be the odours of foetid, dirty, unpleasant or cadaverous things, and noxious fumes and gases. Non-use is to smell nothing at all.

Any excessive intake of a particular taste, or taking foods without regard to prescribed regimens, or not using the sense of taste at all would constitute unhealthy use of the gustatory sense.

Taking excessive numbers of hot or cold baths, receiving massage and oil on the body in excess of the prescribed measure, contact with rough surfaces, unclean objects, harmful objects or very hot or cold objects constitutes insalubrious use of the tactile sense.

Influences of Time and Season (Kala-parinama)

There are activities appropriate for each part of the day, year and age throughout one's life. Disregard of these cycles can be detrimental to one's health and include: daytime sleep (unless prescribed), vigorous physical or mental activity after sunset, sexual activity at the hour of sunrise or sunset or during menstruation, excessive exposure to heat in the winter, cold in the summer, or rain in a non-rainy season.

The Three Causes of Disease

1. *Misuse of the Mind and Body (Prajnaparadha)*
   Supression of natural urges
   Excessive stimulation of natural urges
   Overindulgence in sexual activity
   Poor conduct; immodest behaviour
   Lack of respect for teachers/elders
   Enjoyment of harmful objects
   Using inappropriate force
   Friendship with those who commit evil acts
   Neglect of healthy activities
   Anger, fear, vanity, greed, hatred, intoxication,
     lies, disregard of local customs

2. *Unhealthy Association of the Sense Organs*
   with Sense Objects (Asatmyendriyartha Samyoga)
   Over-, under- and non-stimulation of the five sense organs
   Gazing at very bright objects
   Seeing things that are deformed, alarming, shocking, terrifying
   Not using the eyes
   Hearing loud noises, piercing cries, harsh language, news of deaths,
      insults, untruthful sounds
   Very unpleasant odours, noxious fumes, cadaverous odours
   Excessive intake of any one taste, poorly prepared foods

3. *Vagaries of Time and Season (Kala-Parinama)*
   Disregard for natural cycles
   Daytime sleep (unless prescribed)
   Vigorous exercise after sunset
   Sexual activity during sunrise/sunset/menstruation
   Excessive exposure to heat/winter; cold/summer
   Excessive numbers of hot/cold baths, contact with rough surfaces,
      unclean, harmful, very hot/cold objects

AGENTS OF HEALTH AND DISEASE:
DOSHAS, AMA AND AGNI

These three causative factors can lead to two consequences: they
may cause imbalance in the tridosha or they may diminish agni,
the digestive fire. The latter will result directly in the formation
of ama, incompletely digested food mass. Very often both of
these actions will occur simultaneously. As we saw in Chapter 4,
ama is a white, sticky substance which obstructs the flow of vital
energies, nutrients and wastes through their appropriate channels
(srotas). Thus the vitality and function of the various tissues will
be impaired, influencing the entire human organism.

Since each of the seven dhatus (tissues) are energetically
linked together, impairment in one can easily result in disrupted
function in the others. This is especially true for the chronic
diseases in which agni's function is greatly retarded.

At times it is difficult to establish the causal relationship
between the vitiation of the doshas and the formation of ama
because of decreased agni. In other words, we sometimes cannot
say which process occurs first, nor is it of any great significance.
Aggravated doshas may cause an obstruction of a juxtaposed srota
leading to suppressed agni and ama formation. Or ama formation

may be primary, resulting in a disturbance of the doshas and diminished agni. Regardless of the cause and effect relationship, all diseases have the simultaneous presence of imbalanced doshas, ama formation, obstructed srotas and vitiated dhatus. These factors taken together are the agent of all disease.

THE SIX STAGES OF MANIFESTATION OF DISEASE (SATA KRIYAKALA)

The process through which a disease manifests can be understood in an uncomplicated manner. Due to inappropriate use of the intellect, emotions, diet, lifestyle, sense organs, climate, etc., the doshas become imbalanced. This results in diminished agni, (biological fire) which leads to ama formation (incompletely digested food mass). Ama, together with the vitiated doshas, obstructs the proper flow of nutrients and energies through the srotas (channels) and causes the accumulation of ama. This results in the manifestation of a disease. Ayurveda recognizes six stages in the course of a disease which describe the disruption and evolution of the aggravated doshas.

The six stages are given the name of *sata kriyakala* which means 'six-runged ladder'. Allopathic doctors only first recognize the presence of a disease after stage four in the Ayurvedic system has begun; they then try to institute treatments of the already manifest disease. Ayurvedic practitioners recognize a disease in stages one, two, or three, and by commencing treatment early in the disease process, greatly improve the chance of recuperation. The six stages of disease are:

1. Accumulation (*sancaya*)
2. Aggravation (*prakopa*)
3. Dispersion (*prasara*)
4. Relocation (*sthana samsraya*)
5. Manifestation (*vyakti*)
6. Maturation (*bheda*)

Accumulation (Sancaya)

In this first stage, the doshas begin to accumulate in their own natural sites: vata in the colon, pelvic cavity and bones; pitta in the ileum, jejunum, liver and blood; kapha in the stomach, chest and secretions. Sancaya can be recognized by an observant witness. Accumulated vata creates a sensation of mild distension in the lower abdomen, a tendency towards constipation, increased gas content in the colon, dryness, aversion to cold, mid-afternoon fatigue and a sense of non-specific fear.

Accumulated pitta produces a loss of the natural lustre of the skin, burning sensations throughout the body, hyperacidity especially late at night, increased heat without fever, a desire for cool things and increased irritability.

Kapha accumulation creates lethargy, heaviness, decreased appetite, mild bloating and decreased strength.

Aggravation (Prakopa)

This second stage sees the dosha or doshas which began to accumulate in sancaya become intensely irritated. The irritated doshas are still in their original sites and have not extended to adjacent tissues. Prakopa symptoms are observed more easily than those of sancaya. Vata causes abdominal gas and distension, constipation, intermittent abdominal pains and decreased appetite.

Pitta causes burning pains in the epigastric area, acid reflux, constant thirst and sleeping difficulties.

Kapha manifests as nausea, difficulty waking in the morning, irregular appetite and indigestion.

Dispersion (Prasara)

In this third stage, the aggravated doshas can no longer be contained by their sites of origin and start to flood into the tissues of the body. They first enter the blood which carries them in any direction which offers the least resistance. Dispersion can also occur by direct extension of the excited doshas into nearby organs and malas (waste materials). In addition there is usually a progression of the symptoms at the original site.

At this stage vata reveals itself in continued abdominal pain associated with constipation, headaches, anxiety, abdominal spasms, eczema, dry skin, joint stiffness, lower back pain, pronounced fatigue and insomnia. Pitta causes high fevers, diarrhoea, a burning sensation in the abdomen, rashes, inflammatory bowel symptoms, foul body odour and vomiting. Kapha causes an increase in mucus secretions, bronchitis, asthma, lymphadenitis, depression, nausea and swollen joints sometimes associated with low-grade fevers.

Relocation (Sthana Samsraya)

The fourth stage, sees the accumulation of the aggravated doshas in new sites where they begin to produce clear signs of dysfunction. This is often the stage at which patients are finally motivated to seek medical attention from allopathic physicians. The tissues which are affected may have been predisposed to disease by previous doshic imbalance or injury. The doshas now become firmly anchored in these tissues and the channels which nourish them and remove wastes.

Manifestation (Vyakti)

This stage includes symptoms which can be easily recognized and are grouped by allopathic medicine into specific diseases such as hypertension, diabetes, gout, cholecystitis, etc. There are, in addition to somatic symptoms, psychological phenomena which represent the mental aspect of the same process. These psychological phenomena are thoughts, ideas, emotions and desires, which are present in all earlier stages of the disease as well.

Maturation (Bheda)

In the last stage of disease, the unique complications are fully developed. During this stage, the impact of the disease on the life of the individual is determined. For example, in diabetes mellitus the possibilities are: re-establishment of glucose control, complications (renal failure, diabetic retinopathy, foot ulcerations, cataracts, etc.), further diseases (depression, malabsorption), chronic stable disease (insulin-dependent diabetes mellitus) or death.

THE THREE COURSES OF DISEASE

According to the movement of the imbalanced doshas through the body, three courses of disease have been identified: internal, external and middle. The internal course includes the entire digestive tract, called the *mahasrota* (*maha* – 'great'; *srota* – 'channel'). The middle course includes the tissues of muscle, ligament, tendon, fat, bone, bone marrow, nerve and vital organs. It is called the middle course because these tissues lie between the internal and external courses. The external course includes the plasma, serum, blood cells, skin, nails, hair and superficial tissues.

Examples of internal course diseases are diarrhoea, colitis, constipation, abdominal tumours, liver diseases and malabsorption. Those occurring in the middle course include arthritis, fever, seizure disorders, muscle spasm, sinusitis, coronary artery disease, headache, pancreatitis and osteoporosis. External course diseases are seen with acne, boils, granuloma, haemorrhoids, many chronic skin conditions, erysipelas and some fevers.

We have seen that the cause of a disease is always related to a denial of, or turning away from, natural patterns of living, whether these be in the physical, mental or spiritual realms. These deviations in turn produce accumulations of specific doshas which can lead to a manifestation of disease. The process described in this chapter is the same for all diseases, but varies according to the doshas, the stages, the course taken and the ultimate site where the manifestation occurs. Through its understanding of this process, Ayurveda allows us to treat the disease with appropriate measures at its root.

6

Treatment of Disease

O God, grant us of boons the best, a mind to think, a smiling
love, abundant wealth, a healthy body, speech that is winsome
and days that are fair.

                                                        Rig Veda II, 21:6

CENTURIES AGO IT was understood that the nature of reality is
all-embracing – consisting of God, man, and the universe
all intimately connected. Reality is not a solely divine affair, nor
is it a purely human endeavour, nor a blind cosmic process; it
is divine, human and cosmic all in one. Further, each aspect
of reality is a correlate of the others and all are intimately
connected. Man is a living reflection of the whole of reality;
in man is contained the whole, although in a rather limited
physical package. This knowledge that the individual is nothing
less than a microcosm of the entire universe is essential to an
understanding of the Ayurvedic treatment of disease.

All things present in the macrocosm (the universe) are present
in the microcosm (the individual). Both have a source – the Self
or Creative Principle. Both have a life span and a dissolution;
both have rhythms and cycles. Understanding the unity that
exists between the individual and the universe, the human and
the divine, the material and the spiritual, is itself an important
element in maintaining health. By establishing harmony between
the cycles of the individual and those of nature, we can achieve
freedom from disease, happiness, and even realization of our
true nature.

Ayurveda recognizes that life is a dynamic situation that must be continuously maintained in a state of balance through our own actions, guided by our wisdom regarding man and his relation to the universe. We must take a look around us and acknowledge the daily, monthly and seasonal cycles of which we are a part. We must even realize that we live our lives in relation to both the grandest cycle of expansion and contraction of the universe and to the most fleeting cycle of the tiniest subatomic particle whose vibration exists for perhaps only a billionth of a second. Using Ayurvedic approaches to health, we are able to harmonize our personal life cycles with the other cycles of nature occurring around us. This emphasis on continuous adaptation allows the individual to live a genuinely natural life, free from disease.

Even when we are in excellent health, the daily functioning of our physiologies causes minor imbalances in the doshas. The doshas can be further aggravated by many factors, including inappropriate diet, climate, seasons and emotions. This causes weakening of agni, the digestive fire, which eventually gives rise to unnatural conditions in the body which we recognize as disease. Ayurvedic medicine provides simple preventative methods which re-establish balance at the doshic level quickly and easily. Agni remains high and the body and mind clean and free from disease. There are also measures which may be effectively employed to treat disease states which have already taken root in the physiology.

This chapter is an exploration of the various methods of treatment which Ayurveda has to offer. It includes discussions of both prevention and treatment. Each form of therapy is concisely explained, but you should be aware that volumes could be dedicated to every Ayurvedic treatment under discussion.

MEDITATION

Of all the many forms of treatment described in the Ayurvedic texts, there is one which holds a pre-eminent position – the practice of meditation. This is the fertile soil upon which all other forms of therapy take root. Strictly speaking, without meditation the true healing potential of Ayurvedic medicine cannot be realized.

Meditation is a technique which allows the human mind to

settle into a state of profound stillness while remaining awake and to experience a simple and unlimited state of awareness which is different from our usual waking, dreaming or sleeping states of consciousness. During meditation, the attention is turned inward towards the very source of thought. This can result in a very great expansion of consciousness through the merging of the mind into that limitless, ever-present field which underlies all existence. Many names and descriptions have been given to this all-pervading presence, which is the source of all thought and of all that exists. Some refer to it as the Self, others as Pure Consciousness, and still others as the Unified Field. Perhaps it is best left without a name for it is, in reality, indescribable.

The ancient founders of Ayurveda realized that the most profound perceptions about the nature of man and of reality come not through logic but from *direct experience*. The truths of Ayurveda were realized through intuition rather than through empirical sensory experience. When the physical body is at rest, the senses detached from the sense objects, and the mind in an unattached state, a tremendous flow of energy becomes available. This energy can raise the level of our consciousness and enliven our powers of intuition. We can become aware of personal and universal dynamics which were previously unknown to us. People such as Mozart and Newton no doubt experienced this direct and complete insight when they composed symphonies or understood the laws of science.

According to Ayurveda, it is this direct experience of pure consciousness, the unmanifest source of all that is manifest, that is the fundamental prerequisite for health and healing. This experience of pure consciousness can be accessed through meditation. Over the centuries great sages have discovered truths and practical techniques, and have passed these down to their disciples. That which has proven to be true has survived to the present day; that which was untrue eventually disappeared. This is how the creation works.

The practice of meditation is simple. There are no prerequisites for learning it other than receiving the instruction of a qualified teacher of an authentic form of meditation. A certain amount of desire and enthusiasm is also useful. An experienced Ayurvedic physician can direct you to an appropriate teacher of meditation.

DIET

The digestive system is often regarded as a thirty-six foot long tube through which food passes and where it is made available to the body. This view again highlights our narrow appreciation of our own bodies. In fact, the digestive system is one of the most important communication areas between our internal and external environments. It is a richly innervated system with complex local and systemic nervous and hormonal activities. The degree of intelligence and coordination demonstrated by this area of the body is astounding and it generally runs itself quite well without our conscious involvement.

Ayurveda tells us that, to a large degree, our health and well-being depend on how well our digestive system provides nutrition for the physical body. This is determined not only by which substances we happen to place in our mouths, but also by how well those substances are processed and assimilated. In truth we are not what we eat, as the old adage goes, but what we assimilate.

In addition to its assimilative function another important activity of the digestive tract is elimination. Not all consumed matter is digestible, and some needs to be eliminated, as does the body's copious amounts of endogenous wastes. Ayurveda places great emphasis on the condition of the bowels and the state of the stools, as this can greatly affect the entire physiology.

There is also a constant interaction between the mind and the digestive system. The emotions commonly influence both the function and the structure of the digestive tissues, and vice versa. There is often an immediate digestive response to fear, agitation, infatuation, nervousness or any form of stress. To approach dietetics from an Ayurvedic perspective these psychophysiological connections must always be borne in mind.

According to Ayurveda, diet should be chosen according to the season, the constitution of the individual and the specific doshic imbalances which are present. Many books on Ayurveda promote diets based only on constitutional type, but all three factors must be considered. If an individual is healthy or suffers from only modest imbalances, the diet should reflect the current season with some modifications according to the constitution.

The accompanying tables provide lists of foods that are generally reccommended for each season. Kapha season includes the spring months (mid-March to mid-June in the northern hemisphere, mid-September to mid-December in the southern), pitta season the summer months (mid-June to mid-October in the northern hemisphere, mid-December to mid-April in the southern), and vata season the autumn and winter (mid-October to mid-March in the northern hemisphere, mid-April to mid-September in the southern). In addition to the specific foods included in these tables, other dietary considerations are regarded as equally important:

- Meals should be freshly prepared and warm whenever possible.
- Meals should contain at least a small amount of all six of the basic tastes.
- Do not eat until the previous meal has been completely digested.
- Meals should be eaten with attention and without excess talk.
- Do not eat when nervous, angry or in a highly emotional state.
- Avoid distractions such as reading, television or loud noises during meals; soft, soothing music is acceptable.
- Do not eat if you are thirsty; do not drink if you are hungry.
- Chew each mouthful well before swallowing.
- Do not drink large amounts of water or other liquids before, during or after meals; sipping water during meals is advised.
- The largest, richest meal of the day should be lunch, at approximately 12 noon to 1 pm; dinner should be lighter and no later than 7.30 pm.
- Whenever possible, a twenty-minute walk after dinner is advised.
- Use appropriate spices with meals to promote digestion.
- Meals should be presented in a manner which stimulates both eye and palate.

The following lists of foods are not meant to be exhaustive and reflect foods which are appropriate for most individuals for each season. Through knowledge and reflection upon the principles of rasa, virya, vipaka, and the tridosha, foods which do not appear on these lists can be easily assigned to their proper places.

Constitutional type and specific doshic imbalances must also be considered, so an Ayurvedic practitioner or other competent professional should be consulted for complete dietary guidance.

Kapha Diet (Spring)

Most people will require decreased quantities of food no earlier than 10am and no later than 6pm. Heavy meals in the evening are discouraged. Healthy people should fast one day per week. Favour the pungent, bitter and astringent tastes.

Dairy	*Sweetners*	*Oils*	*Grains*	*Beans*
Goat's milk	Honey	Sunflower	Buckwheat	Aduki
Soy milk		Safflower	Barley	Soy
Low-fat cow's milk		Mustard	Corn	Lima
			Millet	Lentils
			Rye	Tofu
			Quinoa	
			Basmati rice	

Fruits		*Vegetables*		*Nuts/Seeds*
Pomegranates	Broccoli	Artichokes	Onions	Sunflower
Persimmons	Cabbage	Asparagus	Squash	Pumpkin
Cranberries	Carrots	Chilis	Beetroot	Walnuts
Pears	Celery	Radishes	Lettuce	
Apples	Potatoes	Spinach	Cauliflower	
Kiwi fruit	Salads	Sprouts	Green peppers	
Dried fruits	Peas	Alfalfa	Raw vegetables	
Grapefruit	Turnips	Watercress	Chard	
Coconuts	Parsley			

Spices/Herbs	*Beverages*	*Animal Products*
All except salt	Vegetable juices	Chicken (white meat)
	Warm water	Turkey (white meat)
	Spice teas: clove, ginger, cinnamon, dandelion, chicory root	

Pitta Diet (Summer)

Foods should be mostly warm to cool rather than steaming hot:
Favour the sweet, bitter and astringent tastes; cook sparingly
with cheese, yoghurt, tomatoes, lemon or pungent spices and
start and end meals with sweet-tasting foods.

Dairy	Sweetners	Oils	Grains	Beans
Milk	All except	Coconut	Basmati rice	All
Ghee	honey and	Safflower	Wheat	
Butter	molasses	Canola	Barley	
Cream		Sunflower	Quinoa	
Ricotta cheese		Olive	Oats	
Cottage cheese			Short-grain	
Ice cream			brown rice	
Kefir				

Fruits		Vegetables		Nuts/Seeds
Grapes	Oranges	Broccoli	Lettuce	Sunflower
Cherries	Prunes	Cauliflower	Okra	Pumpkin
Plums	Cranberries	Courgettes	Green beans	Almonds
Melons	Figs	Asparagus	Peas	Cashews
Apples	Dates	Cabbage	Cucumber	(unsalted)
Pomegranates	Peaches	Potatoes	Parsnips	
Pineapples	Avocadoes	Aubergine	Beetroot	
Pears	Dried fruits	Sprouts	Green leafy	
Mangoes	Persimmons	Celery	vegetables	
Coconuts	Bananas	Brussel sprouts		

Spices/Herbs		Beverages	Animal Products
Coriander	Cardamom	Sweet fruit	Chicken
Cilantro	Fennel	juices	Turkey
Cinnamon	Nutmeg	cool water	
Dill	Basil	Teas: mint,	
		comfrey, dandelion,	
		alfalfa, hibiscus,	
		kukicha	
		Milk; milkshakes	

Vata Diet (Autumn/Winter)

Most people should consume increased quantities of food. Favour the sweet, sour and salty tastes; warm, well-cooked, oily foods are best.

Dairy	*Sweetners*	*Oils*	*Grains*	*Beans*
All	Cane sugar	All	Basmati rice	Mung dahl
	Honey		Short-grain	Tofu
	Molasses		brown rice	Lentils
	Maple syrup		Wheat	
			Oats	
			Rye	
			Couscous	

Fruits		*Vegetables*		*Nuts/Seeds*
Avocadoes	Pineapples	Sweet potatoe	Peas	All
Mangoes	Olives	Yams	Beetroot	
Papayas	Lemons	Watercress	Carrots	
Grapes	Limes	Asparagus	Turnip	
Peaches	Melons	Green beans	Aubergines	
Cherries	Strawberries	Artichokes	Squash	
Figs	Raspberries	Tomatoes	Peppers	
Coconuts	Bananas	Okra		
Oranges	Apricots			

Spices/Herbs		*Beverages*	*Animal Products*
Ginger	Black pepper	Warm milk	Chicken
Cardamom	Sea salt	Fruit juices	Turkey (white
Cinnamon	Nutmeg	Vegetable juices	meat)
Cumin	Turmeric	Spice teas	Fish
Coriander	Basil	Warm water	Eggs
Horseradish	Cloves		
Asafoetida	Garlic		
Fennel	Fenugreek		

ABHYANGA (SELF-MASSAGE)

One of the salient features of life is that our bodies are constantly changing – life modifies structure continuously. This is clearly seen during the development of the human embryo where a fertilized egg is formed from a sperm and ovum. This single cell forms a multi-celled organism, then a structure with a discernible head and a primitive nervous system, then a foetus with limbs and functioning organ systems. After nine months the process has reached the stage of a mature human foetus. This process of change continues over our entire lifetime – as can be seen, for example, from photographs taken of a person at various stages over a period of fifty years. But although the body is constantly being created and destroyed, and is in fact a totally new body every several years, there is something that connects these bodies and gives each person his or her personality and unique identity. Ayurveda has a name for this connecting factor: *smirti* or memory.

According to Ayurveda our recent and distant past lives and experiences can be observed in the present structure of our bodies. We are also told that this same record of our past experiences can be observed in our minds. The chronicle of our past emotional pleasures and displeasures can be read in our physical form. If, for example, we have led lives of fear we may well have developed a slumped, kyphotic posture and shallow respiratory patterns. Similarly, physical patterns can be seen with anger, greed and all other human feelings if they dominate someone's emotional ground.

By unconsciously holding our bodies in various unnatural postures we may limit the free flow of prana, or vital energy, which by its nature seeks to expand and grow, or else permit it to escape too freely. In the first instance the body is too constricted and solid, in the second too expanded and porous. In either case the mind-body will become disorganized and detached from the guiding wisdom of natural law.

The ancient Ayurvedic sages discovered points distributed throughout the body through which prana must appropriately flow for health to be maintained. These are known as marma points, and there are 107 of them in the human body. According to the Sushruta Samhita, marma points are anatomical regions where two or more of the following structures are present: *sira* (blood vessels), *asthi* (bone and nerve), *snayu* (ligament), *mamsa* (muscle) and *sandhi* (joints). In addition, a marma point is a concentrated point of prana, injury to which can lead to severe disability and even death. Another point of view expressed by Ayurveda is that the marma points are seats of vata, pitta, kapha, rajas, tamas, and sattwa (the three bodily doshas and the subtle

85

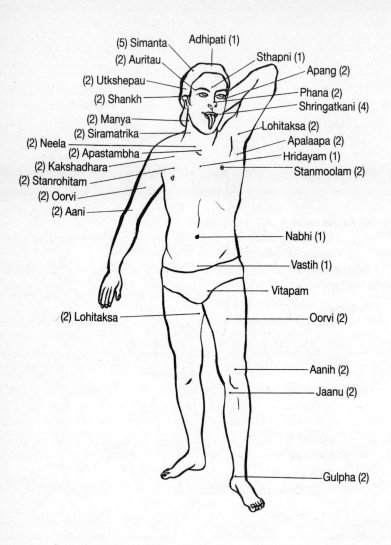

The Marma Points – Front

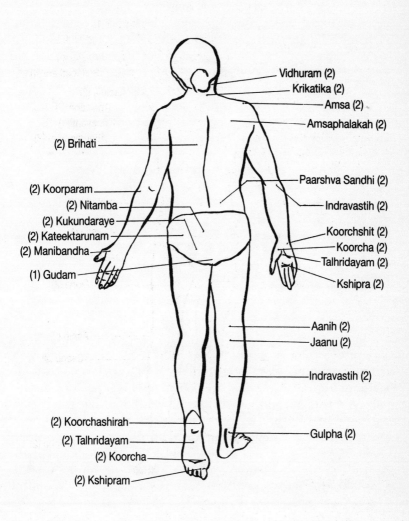

The Marma Points – Back

gunas or energies) and as such are points with substantial effects on both mind and body.

If the flow of prana through one or more marma points is in some way disrupted, disease will manifest. Through memory of past emotional experiences we sometimes adopt postures and physical behaviours which do just that.

Ayurveda has developed a science of massage to unblock and balance the flow of prana through the marma points. These massages are performed with oils which vary according to each individual's constitution and/or particular imbalances. The following chart gives a general indication of which oils are appropriate for each constitution.

Abhyanga Oils for Each Constitutional Type

Vata	*Pitta*	*Kapha*
sesame	coconut	sesame
olive	sandalwood	safflower
almond	pumpkin seed	mustard
amla	almond	corn
bala	sunflower	
wheatgerm		
castor		

Preparing for Self-Massage

Before beginning self-massage one should always lie quietly for a few minutes and take several deep breaths. This is very important. During this relaxation period, the oil can be warming up; set a container of it in hot water before you lie down. The oil only needs to be a few degrees warmer than the skin temperature, about 102–105°F (39–41°C). A few drops of oil should then be applied to the hands and the palms vigorously rubbed together; this energizes the hands and also creates warmth. The self-massage can now proceed.

Self-Massage Technique

There are many traditional Ayurvedic massage techniques which are indicated for various different disorders and doshic predominances. The one presented here is appropriate for all seasons and constitutions and is designed to enhance the immune system and to stimulate the lymphatic and blood circulation. The recommended duration is fifteen to twenty minutes.

Begin by pouring about one-eighth of a cup of oil on the head and massaging vigorously in a 'back and forth' motion, using the ball of the palm. A small amount of oil should then be applied to the nostrils and ears. Proceed to the neck, which should first be rubbed up and down and then gently kneaded. The throat is massaged only in an upward direction and the face is gently rubbed with the palm in a friction-producing motion.

In general the long bones of the body, such as those of the arms and legs, should be given an 'up and down' massage, while the large joints, like the shoulders, elbows and knees, should be massaged in a circular fashion, although it is perfectly acceptable to include some degree of kneading and squeezing. The chest and abdomen should both be massaged in a clockwise direction using the palm. The hips and buttock areas should receive both 'up and down' and circular massage. The hands and feet should receive particular attention. Begin in the centre of the palm or sole, where there are many marma points. Knead these areas well before proceeding to the dorsal aspects (backs) of the hands and feet.

During the massage, always remember that you are providing yourself with nourishment and vitality. Massage, above all else, involves the movement of energies throughout the body. Bear in mind the benefits of what you are doing. Remember that massage cleanses the body, helps to eliminate toxins, opens the srotas (channels) so that energies can flow freely through them and through the marma points, and in doing all this, rejuvenates the mind-body. After completing your massage, lie quietly for a short time.

HERBAL THERAPIES

The ancient Ayurvedists understood that consciousness permeates all forms of life. All that exists is endowed with consciousness and everything in existence plays a unique part in the creation. All life is interconnected and integrated – a synergistic expression of mutual support and nourishment. These vaidyas (master physicians) understood that the apparent multiplicity of life is only an illusion and that, in truth, only the One Self exists.

Entities from all kingdoms – animal, vegetable and mineral – manifest different aspects of the Oneness. Each kingdom exists to receive, transmute and transmit the various forms of energies which exist in the universe. Plants, through the process of photosynthesis, receive light energy from the sun, transmute it into chemical energy in the molecular bonds of carbohydrates, and finally transmit this energy to the animal world as food. Every herb, every plant, can have a unique enlivening effect on our consciousness. But in order for the energies of herbs to become available to us, we must respect and acknowledge their consciousness. We must learn, as the ancient physicians did, to listen to the sacred stories of the herbs as if from the mouths of our most revered sages.

Because of space constraints we cannot cover the entire panorama of Ayurvedic herbal medicine here. What follows therefore is just a survey of some of the more common and time-tested herbal approaches to specific conditions. Do not be too distracted by the manner of presentation; remember that Ayurveda recognizes the human being as a trinity of body, mind and spirit, and herbs work with this whole being and not just with specific symptoms. They do manifest some actions through biochemical and biophysical interactions but they do so in a way that enlivens the entire physiology by augmenting the flow of prana, the vital energy.

Always consult a qualified practitioner for complete information regarding specific herbs for your condition, the dosage, the method of administration and appropriate supporting therapies. Every true Ayurvedic practitioner will be familiar with these three principles of herbal therapeutics:

- Whenever possible use herbs that are indigenous to the region; or country. In any region there are twenty or thirty important herbs that can be used to treat most of the illnesses which manifest there.
- Use mild herbs with gentle physiological actions. Herbs are viewed as bridges between the internal and external cosmic energies which facilitate harmony between the two.
- Always use herbs in conjunction with meditation, diet and other Ayurvedic approaches to health. Without the holistic support of other approaches, very little if any benefit can be expected from herbal therapies.

Unless otherwise indicated the following dosages apply to all of the herbal remedies listed, and they should be used three times a day:

- Infusion: one teaspoon per cup; steep 20 minutes.
- Decoction (for hard and woody substances): two teaspoons per cup; boil over low flame for 20 minutes.
- Powder: three '00' capsules.

Common Ayurvedic Herbal Remedies

Abscess

Powder: marshmallow root, myrrh, echinacea, garlic
Infusion: echinacea, fenugreek, cleavers, cayenne (pinch)

Acne

Infusion: echinacea, wild indigo, dandelion, burdock
Poultice: ½ teaspoon each of sandalwood, turmeric, and myrrh powders mixed with sufficient aloe vera gel to make a paste; apply to area and leave on for 30 minutes; rinse with warm water

Arthritis (early)

Infusion: black cohosh, guaiacum, prickly ash bark, parsley, ginger root.
Poultice: lobelia, cayenne, and cardomom powders mixed with sufficient honey and clove oil to make a paste

Anxiety

Powder: valerian, skullcap, poppy seed, St John's wort
Infusion: gotu kola, valerian, skullcap, mistletoe, peppermint

Asthma

Infusion: elecampane root, lobelia, wild cherry, osha root, comfrey

Back Pain

Decoction: uva ursa, marshmallow root, ginger root, juniper berries

Poultice: cayenne, ginger and mugwort powders mixed with sufficient eucalyptus oil to make a paste

Boils

Infusion: echinacea, blue flag, garlic, myrrh, ginger

Poultice: turmeric, ginger and comfrey powders mixed with sufficient hot water to form a paste

Bronchitis

Infusion: elecampane, coltsfoot, echinacea, black pepper

Decoction: liquorice root, horseradish, ephedra, clove, bloodroot

Powder: echinacea, mullein, osha root, lobelia

Burns

Poultice: St John's wort, comfrey, basil and aloe vera gel mixed with sufficient coconut oil to make a paste

Common Cold

Infusions: a. ginger, cinnamon, liquorice, echinacea
b. echinacea, goldenseal, angelica, ginger, dandelion
c. fresh ginger or fresh peppermint

Constipation

Infusions a. (moderate): i. liquorice root, ginger, cascara sagrada
ii. rhubarb root, liquorice, psyllium husk
b. (mild): 2 teaspoons ghee and 1 teaspoon cinnamon added to 1 cup warm milk; drink 2–3 cups/day

Cough

Decoction: elecampane, wild cherry bark, ground ivy, liquorice root, lobelia, osha root

Infusion: comfrey, bayberry bark, liquorice root, clove; sweeten
with honey
Powder: mullein, goldenseal, coltsfoot, yerba santa

Depression

Infusion: St John's wort, gotu kola, ginko, ginseng root,
skullcap

Diarrhoea

Infusions: i. bayberry bark, catnip, ginger, nutmeg
ii. oak bark, agrimony, coriander

Earache

Infusion: pennywort, mullein, liquorice
3–5 drops of garlic juice in the affected ear

Eczema

Infusion: goldenseal, yellow dock, cleavers, nettles, burdock

Flatulence

Infusions: a. fennel, ginger, anise seed, cardomom
b. calamus root, ginger, angelica, cayenne

Gall Stones

Infusion: dandelion root, fennel, milk thistle, vervain

Gastritis

Infusion: marshmallow, goldenseal, slippery elm, gentian root

Headache (tension)

Infusion: skullcap, valerian, peppermint, rosemary, feverfew
Poultice: ginger powder mixed with sufficient sandalwood oil to
make a paste; apply to forehead and temples

Haemorrhoids

Infusion: liquorice, cascara sagrada, pilewort, marshmallow root, goldenseal
Poultice: witch hazel and goldenseal mixed with sufficient aloe vera gel to make a paste

Hypertension

Infusion: hawthorn berry, yarrow, ginseng root, mistletoe
Powder: maitake mushroom

Influenza

Infusion: goldenseal, echinacea, ginger, cleavers

Insomnia

Infusion (milk): nutmeg, valerian, poppy, passion flower

Kidney Stones

Decoction: corn silk, gravel root, stone root, marshmallow root

Laryngitis

Infusion: balm of Gilead, goldenseal, myrrh, red sage, thyme, bayberry
Gargle: hot water with one teaspoon each of bayberry and red sage

Menstruation

Painful. Infusion: Jamaican dogwood, black cohosh, feverfew, mugwort, valerian, cramp bark
Late. Infusion: pennyroyal, dong quai, parsley, ginger, liquorice root

Excessive. Infusion: raspberry, periwinkle, dong quai, golden-seal

Muscle Spasms

Infusion: valerian, skullcap, ginger, cramp bark, wild yam, Jamaican dogwood

Nausea (non-specific)

Infusion: a. chamomile
b. meadowsweet,
c. peppermint,
d. black horehound.

Phlebitis

Infusion: hawthorn berry, mistletoe, black cohosh

PMS

Infusion: dong quai, mugwort, dandelion, valerian, skullcap

Prostatic Enlargement (Benign Prostatic Hypertrophy)

Infusion: saw palmetto, damiana, juniper berry, poke root

Pharyngitis (sore throat)

Infusion: echinacea, goldenseal, balm of Gilead, horseradish root
Gargle: ¾ glass warm water, ½ teaspoon sage, ½ teaspoon bayberry bark, ¼ teaspoon turmeric

Sinusitis

Infusion: goldenseal, wild indigo, eyebright, ginger, bayberry bark
Inhalation: steam inhalation of eucalyptus leaves and ginger root

Toothache

5 drops clove oil applied to tooth and gums

Ulcer (gastric)

Infusion: slippery elm, meadowsweet, comfrey, gentian, fennel, marshmallow

Ulcer (skin)

Poultice: goldenseal, chapparal, marshmallow in sufficient water to make a paste
Infusion: goldenseal, chickweed, cayenne, comfrey

Varicose Veins (early)

Infusion: juniper berry, thuja leaf, horse chestnut

Vaginitis

Powder: echinacea, goldenseal, juniper berry, oregon grape root, pau d'arco
Douche: decoction of goldenseal, pau d'arco, comfrey, bayberry bark strained and cooled until just warm; add 1½ tablespoons apple cider vinegar and administer as a douche

Weakness (generalized)

Infusion: liquorice, dong quai, ginseng, hawthorn berry, astragalus, wild oats, yellow dock, alfalfa

There are a great many other herbal remedies described in Ayurvedic medicine, as well as a wealth of information regarding the principles of gathering, preparing, combining and administering these substances. The Western 'diagnosis' associated here with each remedy gives only a general indication of possible applications for each group of herbs. Many different conditions can be effectively treated with similar herbs by a knowledgeable practitioner. Always bear in mind that Ayurvedic treatments seek to balance the vital energies, detoxify the physical body and enliven the memory of the One Supreme Self. Diseases are not viewed as separate entities, but only as the consequences of unbalanced doshas.

DINACARYA (DAILY ROUTINE)

Ayurveda places great emphasis on regularity in daily routine. By following a lifestyle which is in harmony with the natural cycle of the day, we reinforce the strength and intelligence already inherent in our physiology. We should adhere to a schedule which includes, for example, the time we rise in the morning, the time we purify and exercise the body, the time we meditate, and the time we take meals. In this way we can protect and nourish our physiology and pursue our lives' highest goals.

We are advised to rise just before sunrise, between 5 am and 6 am, depending on the season. One should then empty one's bladder and bowels, and thus begin the day unburdened by yesterday's wastes. Drinking a glass of tepid water upon rising may help to move the bowels at this early hour if this is not your usual pattern. Next, one should examine and clean the teeth, tongue and face. Toothpastes or powders with pungent, bitter or astringent tastes are recommended. The tongue should be brushed or scraped using a tongue scraper made of gold, silver, tin, or steel.

One should also habitually inhale two drops of anu taila (an Ayurvedic oil) or sesame oil into each nostril every morning. This protects the eyes, nose, and ears from disease and nourishes the ligaments and connective tissues of the head and neck. This practice is also said to strengthen the sense organs, give sweetness and stability to the voice and prevent headaches. Then one should briefly gargle with an appropriate liquid, usually sesame oil. This is nourishing for the teeth and jaws and cleanses the entire supraclavicular lymph node system. This is also the time to trim the nails, and for men to shave.

Next, one should perform abhyanga (self-massage) as described earlier, paying full attention to the technique. If for any reason a full twenty minutes is not available for massage, even a brief period of abhyanga is better than skipping this vital and health-promoting procedure. After removing any excess oil, physical exercise should be done according to constitution and season. Exercise promotes digestion, strength, concentration, lightness, physical comfort and flexibility. But one should never exercise while angry, anxious, exhausted, grieving, laughing or talking. An appropriate form and duration of exercise is best prescribed by an Ayurvedic practitioner on an individual basis. If exercise cannot be taken early in the morning before breakfast, it can be done in the late afternoon before dinner, but not during the evening hours.

After exercise one should bath or shower to remove dirt, perspiration and fatigue, and then put on clean, comfortable clothing. Clean and appropriate dress is said to prevent inauspicious events, and it promotes charm, grace, reputation, confidence and long life. One should then practise meditation, have breakfast and proceed with one's work or study.

After the afternoon activities, the evening should begin with meditation; Ayurveda suggests that the evening meditation begin just before sunset. The evening meal follows; it should be lighter and smaller than the midday meal. A short walk should follow and then some pleasant, light activities. It is best to be in bed before 10 pm, which corresponds to a time in the daily cycle when kapha energy predominates and supports sleep; a new cycle of activity begins with the rise of vata energy between 10 pm and 2 am, and sleep may be less restful then. Proper sleep ensures strength, happiness, virility, and a long life. Ayurveda recognizes the evening hours as the most appropriate for sexual intercourse, which is said to be suitable for married couples only. Intercourse should not occur when the woman is menstruating, or if either partner is impure or is suffering from any kind of infection. Partners should have a passionate desire for each other and neither should be involved with other partners. Sexual practices involving organs other than the genitals are strictly prohibited. Sexual activity is to be avoided during sunrise and sunset, after exercise, during fasts, in places of insufficient privacy and when one has the urge to urinate. Many disease states involve some misuse of sexual energy, which is an important fundamental energy of the emotions. The Ayurvedic sages have a lot to say about the proper management of this vital energy, but a fuller discussion is beyond the scope of this book.

The daily routine described above and summarized below is a classical example suitable for almost everybody. Other practices may be added according to an individual's constitution and doshic imbalances. The daily regimen does not suppress our true nature, but rather enables it to be more freely expressed in all that we think, say and do.

Ayurvedic Daily Routine

- Wake before sunrise.
- Evacuate your bladder and bowels.
- Examine and clean your teeth, tongue, hands, and face.
- Sniff two drops of sesame oil into each nostril.
- Gargle with sesame oil.
- Shave; trim your nails.
- Practise abhyanga (self-massage).
- Take physical exercise appropriate to your condition.
- Bath or shower.
- Dress in clean, comfortable clothing.
- Practise morning meditation (near the hour of sunrise).
- Have a light breakfast.
- Work or study.
- Have your midday meal according to the season and your constitution.
- Continue work or study.
- Practise evening meditation (near the hour of sunset).
- Have your evening meal – lighter, with easily digestible foods.
- Take a short walk.
- Enjoy light, pleasant activities.
- Indulge in sexual intercourse if appropriate.
- Go to sleep before 10 pm.

FASTING

Fasting on one day a week is recommended for the normal, healthy individual. It is an effective initial treatment for many diseases because it both rids the body of toxins and enlivens agni, the digestive fire. During a fast agni is high and since there is no food to digest, it literally begins to burn away toxins in the digestive tract. Many variations of fasts are described in Ayurveda, ranging from the time-honoured water fast to fasts incorporating various juices, teas and broths. Before undertaking a fast of *any* duration it is highly advisable to seek the advice of an Ayurvedic physician or other qualified practitioner.

In addition to the usual twenty-four hour fast once a week, individuals of a kapha constitution may benefit from more prolonged fasting – from three to seven days. Vata and pitta people should generally never exceed three days of fasting. In the case of vata, fasting will aggravate the dosha because of the increase in lightness and air; in pitta individuals prolonged fasting aggravates the fire element, possibly resulting in dizziness, irritability and impatience.

Recommendations for fasts should come from your Ayurvedic practitioner, but here are some commonly prescribed methods.

- Spring or well water
- Single herb teas (ginseng, sassafrass, cardamom, goldenseal, raspberry, ginger)
- Vegetable juices (carrot, beetroot, celery, ginger, kelp)

The amount of liquid taken varies, but in general one should take between 2 and 4 pints (1–2 litres) each day. Fruit juices are discouraged as they tend to form ama when taken during fasts, although lemon juice is an exception to this rule. Certain herbs, we are told, if taken in the form of a tea during a fast, will further assist in the elimination of toxins from the body. These include: black pepper, long pepper (pippili), cayenne, dry ginger, asafoetida, basil and cardamom. Care must be taken, however, by those with a pitta constitution, not to aggravate the pitta, so these herbs are best combined with cooler, bitter herbs, such as barberry, goldenseal, chaparral, gentian, neem or aloe.

As I have said, almost everyone will benefit from a weekly fast. There is often an increase in clarity and lightness, as well as a greater availability of subtle energies to the mind. While you are fasting, pay close attention to your mental and physical energy levels. If you notice an abrupt decrease in these energies, discontinue the fast.

PANCHAKARMA – THE FIVE PURIFICATION THERAPIES

Disease manifests in the human body as a result of the abnormal accumulation of one or more doshas in the tissues. Panchakarma is the therapeutic means by which excess doshic energies are eliminated from the physiology. Panchakarma means 'the five actions', and these actions allude to natural and gentle cleansing actions which normally occur in everyone. Panchakarma therapies merely enliven the body's own natural mechanisms for eliminating toxins.

Nasya

This refers to the administration of substances via the nasal passages to remove excess kapha dosha from the head and supraclavicular (neck) regions.

The sense of smell occurs when molecules of the element earth stimulate receptors within the nostrils. Impulses reach the brain via the olfactory nerve which also carries sensory information to the amygdala and hippocampus – areas of the brain associated with the emotional content of conscious thought. Thus the nasal administration of specific substances can help correct disorders with emotional components. Nasya also helps rid the nose, sinus cavities, throat and head region of accumulated toxins.

There are many different substances used in nasya. The more common ones include calamus root powder, gotu kola powder, ginger powder and various powdered peppers. Also commonly used are ghee, anu oil, aloe vera juice, sesame oil, onion juice, tulsi juice, milk and various herbal extracts. Nasya is contra-indicated during menstruation and pregnancy, as well as after eating, bathing, sexual intercourse or exercise. Besides being a general purification technique, nasya is specifically useful in treating the following disease conditions: sinusitis, laryngitis, tension and migraine headaches, otitis media, eye infections, rhinorrhoea, acne, allergic rhinitis, fatigue, laziness and anxiety.

Vamana

This is vomiting therapy, which is employed to remove excess kapha dosha from the stomach and chest.

In the human embryo the stomach and the lungs arise from the same primitive tissue, the entoderm. Although separated in adults, a subtle connection remains intact between the two organs. Thus, when the stomach is cleansed, so are the lungs. When the glands lining the respiratory tract become hyperactive and cause congestion, asthma, bronchitis and coughing, vamana therapy can help eliminate not only large amounts of mucus secretions, but also kapha itself, which often lies at the root of the condition. Methods of inducing vomiting include drinking five or six cups of the following herbal infusions: lobelia, nux vomica, liquorice, calamus or pennyroyal. Also useful for certain patients are milk, salt water, comfrey and osha root. After taking the prescribed amount of the appropriate emetic patients must gently rub the back of the tongue to induce vomiting. Once the vomitus is expelled you will instantly feel a lightness and clarity, and be relieved from congestion, wheezing and heaviness. You should rest for about thirty minutes after this therapy.

Vamana can be repeated once a day for several days or performed just once with great benefit. It is usually performed on an empty stomach, first thing in the morning. The contra-indications for vamana are old age, weakness, angina, tuberculosis, menstruation, pregnancy and hypertension.

Virechana

This purgative therapy involves the ingestion of an oleating substance followed by a gentle laxative to eliminate excess pitta dosha and cleanse the blood, liver, spleen, small intestine and sweat glands.

There are many excellent herbs which can be used to create the mild laxative effect necessary for this aspect of panchakarma. Commonly used substances are: castor oil, senna leaf tea, aloe vera gel, ghee, triphala, cascara sagrada, rhubarb, dandelion, and psyllium seed infusion. It is often useful if virechana is preceded by several days of *snehana* (ingestion of an unctuous substance), and if hot baths are taken during this period. Contra-indications are fever, abdominal pain, diarrhoea, weakness, Crohn's disease, ulcerative colitis or directly after high colonic therapy.

Basti

This is the application of medicated oils and herbalized decoctions as an enema to remove excess vata dosha from the colon, rectum, lumbosacral region and bones.

The literal meaning of basti is 'urinary bladder'. The procedure which we call enema has become known as basti because the urinary bladders of cows, buffaloes and goats were often used to administer the substances. Vata dosha regulates the elimination of urine, faeces and other wastes and therefore plays a prominent role in the manifestation of disease. Vata is located in the colon, rectum and bones. Medications given via the rectum are considered to be complete treatments for vata disorders as well as being effective for many pitta and kapha disorders as well. There are three main kinds of basti therapies, each useful for different conditions: nutritive, tonifying and reducing.

The substances used for basti vary widely and include mixtures of oils, such as sesame, castor and olive, herbalized oils, decoctions of water or milk (including calamus root, triphala, comfrey, ginger, goldenseal, liquorice, gotu kola) and broths of various meats and bone marrows. Basti is recognized as a very effective treatment for constipation, low back pain, arthritis, anxiety, headache, viral syndromes, sexual dysfunction and many other conditions. It is contra-indicated in the case of shortness of breath, chest pains, rectal bleeding or infection, acute diarrhoea or poorly controlled diabetes mellitus.

Raktamokshana

This therapy involves the removal of small quantities of blood from a vein to eliminate toxins and excess pitta dosha from the blood, lymph and deeper tissues.

Because of its invasive nature, this therapy is used less commonly today than in past times. Blood letting is known to stimulate the immune system and to eliminate toxins which may have accumulated in the vascular channels and deeper tissues. Generally, herbal blood purifiers are an effective alternative approach.

The most commonly used herbs for this purpose are: yellow dock, burdock, goldenseal, thuja, cleavers and red clover. Also useful are turmeric, saffron, sandalwood and calamus root. Indications for blood purification include chronic skin disorders such as acne, eczema, abscess, urticaria, rashes, hepatomegaly, splenomegaly, abdominal tumours, fevers, gout, haemorrhoids, jaundice, proctitis and herpes genitalis. When less invasive measures have been ineffective, removal of a small amount of venous blood may be performed by a physician experienced in this procedure.

In addition to these five primary therapies, Panchakarma includes other treatments which are often added according to an individual's needs. These include:

- *Swedena*: the use of herbalized steam to stimulate the elimination of toxins through the skin
- *Snehana*: the ingestion of oily substances over a period of several days to rid the body of excess vata dosha; often precedes virechana therapy
- *Shirodhara*: the dripping of warm herbalized oil onto the forehead region for various periods of time; the oil drips from a small opening in the bottom of a special pot which is suspended directly over the patient's head
- *Udvartna*: the application of herbal paste to the entire body followed by wrapping in warm blankets, and the subsequent removal of the dried paste using specialized massage techniques
- *Pichhila*: the pouring of warm oil over the body in copious amounts and rhythmically massaging it into the skin

AROMATHERAPY

The essential oils of many plants are used in massage and steam inhalation, or in aroma-diffuser pots to produce odours which have therapeutic effects on the mind and body. Essential oils are highly volatile aromatic oils produced by plants in order to attract insects, to discourage predators or to fight off disease. When molecules of these oils are detected by the human olfactory cells in the nostrils, there is an immediate and profound response in the limbic area of the brain. This area influences our emotions, libido and memory. In Ayurveda, aromas are used to pacify aggravated doshas.

The method of application of aromatherapy is determined by the constitutional type (prakriti) of the individual being treated. Vata individuals respond best to massage techniques which incorporate aroma oils; pitta individuals are most responsive to aroma pot therapy; kapha types are best suited to steam inhalation techniques. However it is clear that all three are effective to some extent for all three prakritis. The following chart illustrates which essential oil aromas are best for each of the three doshas.

Recommended Essential Oils for Pacifying the Three Doshas

Vata	Pitta	Kapha
Lavender	Sandalwood	Eucalyptus
Cedarwood	Rose	Basil
Juniper	Lavender	Tulsi
Ylang-ylang	Gardenia	Rosemary
Patchouli	Saffron	Peppermint
Myrrh	Jasmine	Lemon
Sage	Lotus	Camphor
Geranium	Vetivert	Frankincense
Tulsi		Sage

The massage techniques used require a knowledge of the marma points located throughout the body, which number 107 in all. Each dosha requires the application of an appropriate essential oil and the stimulation of specific groups of marma points when it is in an aggravated state.

Steam inhalation aromatherapy involves the addition of between six and ten drops of essential oil to a medium-sized (approximately 4-pint or 2-litre) pot of boiling water, which is placed on a table. The patient bends over the steaming water containing the aroma oil, drapes a towel over the head and pot to create a 'tent' effect, and breathes in the vapours for 5–15 minutes.

Diffuser or pot-pouri pots are small ceramic vessels, to which hot water and 10–15 drops of essential oil are added. Beneath this vessel is placed a small candle which provides the heat necessary to volatilize the oil gradually into the surrounding air. The pot is usually left to diffuse its aroma into the room for two or three hours.

It is beyond the scope of this brief introduction to to describe some of the more esoteric forms of Ayurvedic treatment, but for the sake of completeness, I will just mention them.

Ayurvedic practitioners are traditionally trained in what we might term climatology, minerology and psychology. They also receive extensive training in the art of predictive astrology or *jyotish.* This often enables the vaidya practitioner to know whether an individual has certain predilections for particular diseases at particular times. The remedies for some of the astrological situations include the use of gems and mantras. These two forms of treatment were part of the Ayurvedic training in ancient times. Today much of this knowledge of the vibratory nature of sounds and crystalline structures has been lost or distorted, but fortunately at least some of it has survived.

Ayurveda also recognizes the value of various yoga *asanas* or postures, as described by Patanjali. This great ancient sage described eight limbs of yogic practices:

- *Yama*: right outer conduct in daily life: non-injury; truthfulness; abstension from stealing, impurity, and covetousness.
- *Niyama*: right inner conduct in daily life: purity and serenity; fervent aspiration and scriptural study; perfect obedience to the Master.
- *Asana*: bodily postures perfected through steady effort.
- *Pranayama*: right breathing.
- *Pratyahara*: attention.
- *Dharana*: concentration.
- *Dhyana*: meditation.
- *Samadhi*: perfect balance.

One could devote lifetimes to understanding the full value of any one of these practices. Our purpose here is to point out that Ayurvedic medicine incorporates the third limb, the asanas, to develop the strength and flexibility of the physical body as well as to promote the unimpeded flow of energies throughout the mind-body. Various postures also help to release and move stagnant energies and impurities which have accumulated in the marma points and chakras. When allowed to remain stagnant these energies often give rise to physical and psychological disorders. There are also specific asanas which are most suitable for individuals of each constitutional type. These should be prescribed individually by an Ayurvedic practitioner completely familiar with the science of yoga asanas and with the medical condition of the patient.

Glossary

Abhyanga: ancient massage using friction
Agni: fire; biological digestive energy
Akasha: space; ether
Akriti: face
Ama: undigested food
Amla: sour
Anupanam: vehicle to carry a herb
Asana: posture in Hatha Yoga
Asthi dhatu: bone tissue
Basti: enema therapy
Bhutagni: energy that works specifically with one of the five elements
Brahma: a Hindu god
Dhatu(s): the seven basic tissues of the physical body
Dhatu agnis: agnis (q.v.) which regulate the physiological processes of each tissue
Dinacharya: daily routine
Dosha: that which darkens; force which governs the physiological processes
Drika: eyes
Guna: quality; subtle energy
Jala: water
Jathara agni: agni (q.v.) which catalyses the production of digestive enzymes
Jihva: tongue
Kapha dosha: bioenergy related to structure and stability
Karma: action
Kasaya: astringent
Katu: pungent
Madhura: sweet

Mahabhutas: the five fundamental elements
Majja dhatu: bone marrow tissue
Mala: waste product of the body
Malam: faeces
Mamsa dhatu: muscle tissue
Manas: the discursive mind
Marma shariram: superficial points of concentrated energy
Meda dhatu: fatty tissue
Mutra: urine
Nadi: pulse
Nasya: the administration of therapeutic substances via the nasal passages
Ojas: vital energy of an individual
Panchakarma: five therapies; profound cleansing techniques
Pichhila: massage with warm oil
Pitta dosha: bioenergy relating to transformation and digestion
Prabhava: special action; unique energy
Prakriti: essential nature of an individual
Prana: breath; subtle energy; Life Force
Pranayama: specialized breathing exercises
Pratyahara: practices which quieten the mind
Prthivi: earth
Purisha: faeces
Purusha: any individual person; an embodied human soul
Rajas: a subtle energy related to movement or activity
Rakta dhatu: blood cells
Rakta mokshana: therapeutic blood letting
Rasa: taste; juice; sap
Rasa dhatu: plasma
Rasayana: strengthening and rejuvenating substance
Sata kriyakala: six stages of disease
Sattwa: a subtle energy related to harmony, balance, and rest
Shabda: voice
Shirodhara: the therapeutic dripping of oil onto the forehead
Snehana: oleation therapy
Sparsa: skin
Srota: channel; vessel; duct
Sukra dhatu: reproductive tissues
Sveda: perspiration
Swedana: perspiration therapy
Tamas: a subtle energy related to inertia
Tejas: fire
Tikta: bitter
Udvartna: the therapeutic application of herbal paste to the body

Vamana: therapeutic vomiting
Vanksana: kidneys
Vata dosha: bioenergy relating to motion, animation, action
Vayu: wind
Vipaka: internal taste of a substance
Virechana: elimination or purging therapy
Virya: potency
Yoga: to unite, connect, yoke (e.g. body and mind)

Useful Addresses

Scott Gerson, MD
International Federation for Ayurveda
Ayurvedic Medicine of New York
13 West Ninth Street
New York, NY 10011
Tel. 212–505–8971

Andrew Weil, MD
1975 West Hunter Road
Tucson, Arizona 85737
Tel. 602–742–6788

American Holistic Medical Association
4101 Lake Boone Trail, Suite 201
Raleigh, North Carolina 27607
Tel. 919–787–5181

Angelica's Traditional Herbs and Foods
147 First Avenue
New York, NY 10003
Tel. 212–677–1549

Aphrodesia Products, Inc.
264 Bleeker Street
New York, NY 10011
Tel. 212–989–6440

Mark Blumenthal
American Botanical Council
PO Box 201660
Austin, Texas 78720
Tel. 512–331–8868

Gaia Herbs
62 Old Littleton Road
Harvard, Massachusetts 01451
Tel. 508–456–3049

Phyto-Pharmica
PO Box 1348
Green Bay, Wisconsin 54305
Tel. 414–435–4200

UK

Dr Nicholas G. Kostopoulos, MD (Ath), MF Hom
354 Finchley Road
London NW3 7AJ

Culpepper Ltd.
21 Bruton Street
London W1X 7DA
Tel. 071–629–4559

AUSTRALIA

Dr Krishna Kumar, MD (Ayu, OIUCM) FIIM
Australian School of Ayurveda
27 Blight Street
Ridleyton, South Australia 5008
Tel. (08) 346–0631

Dr Karl Horst Poehlmann PhD, MBBS
28 Garden Terrace
Underdale, South Australia 5032
Tel. (08) 352–8057

Further Reading

Charaka Samhita, 3 volumes,
Chowkhamba Press,
Varanasi, India, 1983.

Sushruta Samhita, 3 volumes,
Chowkhamba Press,
Varanasi, India, 1981.

Ashtanga Hridayam, 2 volumes,
Krishnadas Academy Publishers,
Varanasi, India, 1981.

Madhava Nidanam,
Chowkhamba Press,
Varanasi, India, 1987.

Sarngadhara Samhita,
Srigokul Mudranalaya,
Varanasi, India, 1984.

Artharva Veda,
Munshiram Manoharlal Publishers, Ltd.,
New Delhi, India, 1982.

Index

abdominal distention 40, 42
abdominal pain 40, 41, 42, 48
abhyanga 84–9, 97, 99
acne 91
agni 33, 46–8, 58, 72–3
  definition 46
  dhatuagni 47
  disorders 46–7
  therapies 58
alochaka pitta 26
aloe vera 91, 92, 94
ama 48–9
amla 60–1, 72–3
anabolism 17, 27
anu taila 97
apana vata 22
appetite, lack of 21
aromatherapy 104–5
arthritis 91
ashwagandha 39
asthi dhatu 36, 38
asthma 91
astrology 106
avalambaka kapha 29

back pain 92
basti 102
bhrajaka pitta 26
bleeding therapy see raktamokshana
bodhaka kapha 29
boils 92
bronchitis 47, 64
burdock 91

burning 36, 41

calamus 93
cardamon 100
castor oil 88, 102, 103
catabolism 17
cayenne 96
Charaka 12
Charaka Samhita 11, 12
coconut oil 88, 92
cold, common 92
colon 21, 40
consciousness 79
constipation 92
corn oil 88
cough 92
cumin 96

daily routine see dinacharya
depression 23, 93
dhatus 34–8
diagnosis 23, 26, 30
diarrhoea 25, 27, 47, 93
diet 80–4
  kapha 82
  pitta 82–3
  vata 83
digestion 25
  disorders 21, 25, 29
  herbs for 26
dinacharya 97–9

113

disease 62–76
  categories 64–5
  causes 70–2
  of the three doshas 65–9
  six stages 73–5
  three courses 75–6
doshas, three 15–32, 33, 49, 50–3, 56

earache 93
eczema 93
elements, five 3–4, 13–15
emotions 85
enemas *see* basti
essential oils 105
exercise 97, 98
eyes 23, 24, 26, 27

faeces *see* purisha
fasting 99, 100
fatigue 32, 38
fear 36, 71
fever 26, 53, 64, 68
flatulence 93

garlic 92, 93
gas *see* flatulence
gastritis 93
ghee 39
gotu kola 93
gunas 53–6

hair 24, 28
headache 93
heart 22, 29
haemorrhoids 94
herbal therapies 89–97
honey 82, 91
humours *see* doshas
hypertension 94

impotence 38
indigestion 94
insomnia 21, 94
intelligence 5, 6, 24
intestines 40

joints 29, 30

kapha 27–30
  attributes 28

constitution 28
diagnosis 30
diet 81
disorders 29
herbs 82
seasons 30, 80–1
seats of *see* subdoshas
subdoshas 29–30
time 30
kidneys 29
kledaka kapha 29

large intestine *see* colon
laxative 92
life style 97
liver 25
lunch 81
lungs 101
lymph 43

majja dhatu 36–7, 38
malas 33, 40–2
mamsa dhatu 35–6, 38
marma points 85–8
massage, self *see* abhyanga
meat 82, 83, 84
meda dhatu 36, 38
meditation 2, 78–9
memory 30
menstruation 44, 45, 94, 95
mental disorders 67
metabolism 17
mind 77–8
mutra 41

nails 38
nasya 101
nausea 38, 95
numbness 36

obesity 28
ojas 37, 39
oil massage *see* abhyanga
oleation therapy *see* snehana

pachaka pitta 25
pain 53, 64, 66
panchakarma 100–4
Pantanjali 106
pitta 23–7
  attributes 24

constitution 24
diagnosis 26–7
diet 82–3
disorders 25
herbs 83
seasons 26, 81
seats of *see* subdoshas
subdoshas 25–6
time 26
prabhava 60–1
prakriti 49–53
prana 43, 44, 57
prana vata 22
purgation therapy *see* virechana
purisha 40–1

rajas 53, 85
rakta dhatu 35
raktamokshana 103
ranjaka pitta 25–6
rasa dhatu 34–5
rasa 56–9
rash 38
reproductive system 37–45
Rig Veda 3, 9

sadhaka pitta 25
samana vata 22
Sanskrit 5, 6
sattwa 53, 85
sesame oil 97
sexual intercourse 98
sexual vitality 37
Self 1, 2, 10, 13, 77
self-realization 11
shatavari 39
sinusitis 95
skin 23, 26, 27, 30
sleep 47
sleshaka kapha 30
small intestine 25
soma 9
sore throat 95
srotas 33, 42–6
stuttering 22

sukra dhatu 37–8
Sushruta Samhita 12
sveda 41
swedana therapy 104

tamas 53, 85
tarpaka kapha 30
tastes, six 56–9
tea 82, 83, 84, 100
tejas 13, 15, 16
thirst 25, 41, 42
tissues *see* dhatus
tongue 28, 49
toxins *see* ama
tridosha 15–32

udana vata 22
ulcers 96
Upanishads 10–11
urine *see* mutra

vamana therapy 101–3
vata 19–23
    attributes 20
    constitution 20
    diagnosis 23
    diet 83-4
    disorders 23
    herbs 84
    seasons 81
    sites of *see* subdoshas
    subdoshas 21–2
    time 23
Vedas 8–11
vipaka 60
virechana therapy 102
virya 59
vyana vata 22

waste products *see* malas
water 97
Western medicine 62–3

Yoga, asanas 106